Complex Cases in Echocardiography

Complex Cases in Echocardiography

EDITOR-IN-CHIEF

Robert J. Siegel, MD

Professor of Medicine
Director, Cardiac Noninvasive Laboratory
Cedars-Sinai Medical Center
Los Angeles, California

ASSISTANT EDITOR

Roy Beigel, MD

The Leviev Heart Center
Sheba Medical Center
Tel Hashomer
Sackler School of Medicine
Tel Aviv University
Tel Aviv, Israel
The Heart Institute
Cedars-Sinai Medical Center
Los Angeles, California

EDITORS

Swaminatha V. Gurudevan, MD

Cardiologist, Division of Cardiology
Cedars-Sinai Medical Center
Los Angeles, California

Takahiro Shiota, MD

Associate Director, Cardiac Noninvasive Laboratory
Cedars-Sinai Medical Center
Los Angeles, California

Kirsten Tolstrup, MD

Assistant Director, Cardiac Noninvasive Laboratory
Cedars-Sinai Medical Center
Los Angeles, California

Nina Wunderlich, MD

Co-Director, CardioVascular Center Frankfurt
Frankfurt, Germany

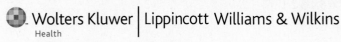

Wolters Kluwer | Lippincott Williams & Wilkins
Health

Philadelphia • Baltimore • New York • London
Buenos Aires • Hong Kong • Sydney • Tokyo

Acquisitions Editor: Julie Goolsby
Product Manager: Leanne Vandetty
Production Project Manager: Priscilla Crater
Senior Manufacturing Coordinator: Beth Welsh
Marketing Manager: Stephanie Manzo
Design Coordinator: Joan Wendt
Production Service: Absolute Service, Inc.

© 2014 by LIPPINCOTT WILLIAMS & WILKINS, a WOLTERS KLUWER business
Two Commerce Square
2001 Market Street
Philadelphia, PA 19103 USA
LWW.com

Printed in China

Library of Congress Cataloging-in-Publication Data

Complex cases in echocardiography / editor-in-chief, Robert J. Siegel ; editors, Swaminatha V. Gurudevan, Takahiro Shiota, Kirsten Tolstrup, Nina Wunderlich ; assistant editor Roy Beigel.
     p. ; cm.
  Includes bibliographical references and index.
  ISBN 978-1-4511-7646-9
  I. Siegel, Robert J., editor of compilation.
  [DNLM: 1. Echocardiography—Case Reports. 2. Echocardiography—Examination Questions. WG 18.2]
  RC683.5.E5
  616.1'207543—dc23

                                  2013026478

Care has been taken to confirm the accuracy of the information presented and to describe generally accepted practices. However, the authors, editors, and publisher are not responsible for errors or omissions or for any consequences from application of the information in this book and make no warranty, expressed or implied, with respect to the currency, completeness, or accuracy of the contents of the publication. Application of the information in a particular situation remains the professional responsibility of the practitioner.

The authors, editors, and publisher have exerted every effort to ensure that drug selection and dosage set forth in this text are in accordance with current recommendations and practice at the time of publication. However, in view of ongoing research, changes in government regulations, and the constant flow of information relating to drug therapy and drug reactions, the reader is urged to check the package insert for each drug for any change in indications and dosage and for added warnings and precautions. This is particularly important when the recommended agent is a new or infrequently employed drug.

Some drugs and medical devices presented in the publication have Food and Drug Administration (FDA) clearance for limited use in restricted research settings. It is the responsibility of the health care provider to ascertain the FDA status of each drug or device planned for use in their clinical practice.

To purchase additional copies of this book, call our customer service department at (800) 638-3030 or fax orders to (301) 223-2320. International customers should call (301) 223-2300.

Visit Lippincott Williams & Wilkins on the Internet at LWW.com. Lippincott Williams & Wilkins customer service representatives are available from 8:30 am to 6 pm, EST.

10 9 8 7 6 5 4 3 2 1

Contributors

Roy Beigel, MD
Cardiology and Internal Medicine
The Leviev Heart Center
Sheba Medical Center
Tel Hashomer, Israel
Visiting Scientist
Cedars Sinai Medical Center
Los Angeles, California

Jacob P. Dal-Bianco, MD
Cardiology Fellow
The Heart Institute
Cedars Sinai Medical Center
Los Angeles, California

Jennifer Franke, MD
Department of Cardiology
University of Heidelberg
Heidelberg, Germany

Swaminatha V. Gurudevan, MD
Associate Clinical Professor of Medicine, UCLA
Assistant Director, Cardiac Noninvasive Laboratory
The Heart Institute
Cedars Sinai Medical Center
Los Angeles, California

Huao Luo, MD, PhD
Clinical and Research Sonographer
The Heart Institute
Cedars Sinai Medical Center
Los Angeles, California

Ryan P. Morrissey, MD
Cardiology Fellow
The Heart Institute
Cedars Sinai Medical Center
Los Angeles, California

Jennifer B. Plotkin
Massachusetts Institute of Technology
Cambridge, Massachusetts

Asim Rafique, MD
Cardiology Fellow
The Heart Institute
Cedars Sinai Medical Center
Los Angeles, California

Takahiro Shiota, MD
Professor of Medicine, Cedars Sinai, UCLA
Associate Director, Cardiac Noninvasive Laboratory
The Heart Institute
Cedars Sinai Medical Center
Los Angeles, California

Robert J. Siegel, MD
Professor of Medicine, Cedars Sinai, UCLA
Kennamer Chair in Cardiac Ultrasound
Director, Cardiac Noninvasive Laboratory
The Heart Institute
Cedars Sinai Medical Center
Los Angeles, California

Nirmal Singh, MBBS
Cedars-Sinai Medical Center
Los Angeles, California

Leandro Slipczuk, MD, PhD
Cardiology Fellow
The Heart Institute
Cedars Sinai Medical Center
Los Angeles, California

Kirsten Tolsrup, MD
Associate Professor of Medicine
Medical Director
Heart Station and Echolab
Division of Cardiology
University of New Mexico Health Sciences
Albuquerque, New Mexico

Janet Wei, MD
Cardiology Fellow
The Heart Institute
Cedars Sinai Medical Center
Los Angeles, California

Nina C. Wunderlich, MD
Cardiovascular Center Darmstadt
Darmstadt, Germany

Parham Zarini, MD
Resident in Medicine
Cedars Sinai Medical Center
Los Angeles, California

Preface

With the numerous and varied echocardiography texts available, why write another book on echocardiography? The authors of this text, all active clinical cardiologists and echocardiologists, present a comprehensive guide to echocardiography in a case-based format, linked to actual patients, ranging from the relevant common case scenarios to diagnostic dilemmas encountered by both clinicians and echocardiologists. We have included a broad spectrum of cardiovascular diseases and echo images that the clinician-echocardiologist will encounter in their clinical practice. Some of the cases are simple; others are more complex. We present cases seen in the performance of emergency as well as intraoperative transesophageal echocardiography (TEE), during real-time echo-guidance of transcatheter interventions, and echocardiograms seen during routine reading in a high-volume echo laboratory. Each case is associated with a series of questions and answers, with reference(s) provided for each case. The web-based portion of this book is an essential component of the case solving process, allowing the reader to "be there for each case" and review the actual case video clips. In addition to cases involving M-mode, 2D, and 3D echo, as well as TEE and Doppler ultrasound, there are cases in which a particular physical finding or electrocardiogram is to be matched with the patient's corresponding echocardiogram.

The varied cases are clinically relevant, interesting, educational, and reflect the writing and teaching style of each individual co-editor. The scope of the material is comprehensive and serves as a dynamic format by which to prepare for the National Board of Echocardiography examinations.

This book and the accompanying web-based series of cases are dedicated to our patients and to our teachers. We hope you find it educational, enjoyable, and helpful.

Contents

Digital Contents

CASE 1

Marfan Syndrome, Status Post Bentall Procedure

A 19-year-old woman with Marfan syndrome is status post Bentall procedure (Figs. 1-1 to 1-4 and Videos 1-1 to 1-4).

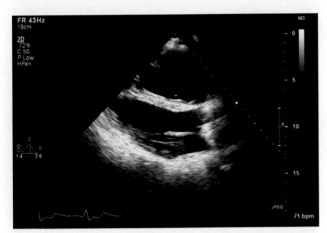

Figure 1-1.

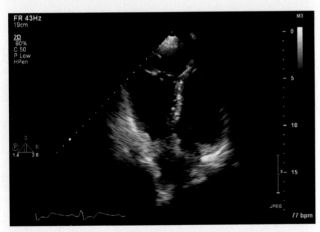

Figure 1-2.

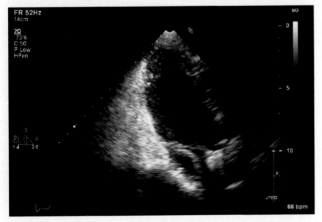

Figure 1-3.

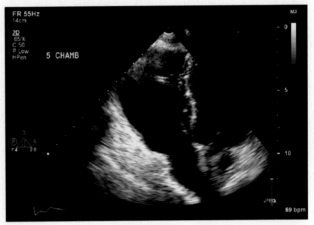

Figure 1-4.

QUESTION 1. What complication occurred during the surgery?

    A. Aortic dissection

    B. Ligation of the left circumflex artery

    C. Occlusion of the right coronary artery (RCA)

    D. Occlusion of the left anterior descending artery

QUESTION 2. The right ventricle (RV) can be identified by:

    A. Smaller size compared with the left ventricle (LV)

    B. Presence of moderator band

    C. Tricuspid annulus superior to the mitral annulus

    D. All of the options

Answers

ANSWER 1: C. Although ligation of the left circumflex artery is a dreaded complication of mitral valve repair/replacement, difficulty with reimplantation of either coronary artery can occur with a Bentall procedure, with occlusion of the RCA being more common. In these images, the RV is thinned and severely dilated, and the inferior wall of the LV is thinned. Both of the findings are consistent with a prior RCA infarction.

Suggested Reading

Salerno TA, Bergsland J, Calafiore AM, et al. Acute right ventricular failure during aortic valvular operation due to mechanical problem in the right coronary artery. *Ann Thorac Surg.* 1996;61: 706–707.

ANSWER 2: B. The RV, although not always the smaller of the two ventricles as in the case of D-transposition of the great vessels, can be correctly identified by the presence of the moderator band. Furthermore, the tricuspid valve morphologically "follows" the RV and can be differentiated from the mitral valve given its more inferior location (it is more apical in the ventricle compared with the mitral valve).

CASE 2

Mild Exertional Dyspnea

A 23-year-old woman has mild exertional dyspnea. Her electrocardiogram is normal, but she has a systolic and diastolic heart murmur. The 2D transesophageal echocardiogram (TEE) images show long-axis (LAX) and short-axis (SAX) views with and without color Doppler (Videos 2-1 and 2-2 and Figs. 2-1 to 2-3).

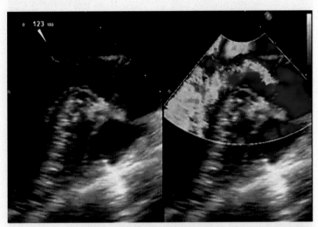

Figure 2-1. TEE 123°, LAX view without and with color Doppler in diastole.

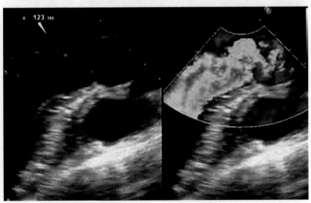

Figure 2-2. TEE 123°, LAX view without and with color Doppler in systole.

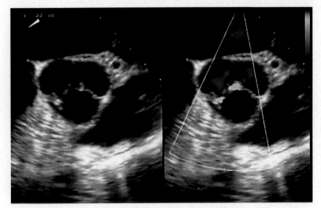

Figure 2-3. TEE 33°, SAX view in diastole.

QUESTION 1. Which diagnoses are correct (select all that apply)?

- A. Severe aortic insufficiency
- B. Mild-to-moderate aortic insufficiency and subvalvular membrane
- C. Aortic cusp prolapse
- D. Subvalvular membrane
- E. Ruptured sinus of Valsalva aneurysm
- F. Endocarditis

QUESTION 2. Associated congenital heart defects are found in 25% to 50% of patients with discrete (or membranous) subvalvular aortic stenosis (DSAS). Which defect is associated with DSAS and needs to be evaluated?

- A. Patent ductus arteriosus, coarctation of the aorta, bicuspid aortic valve, interrupted aortic arch
- B. Ventricular septal defect
- C. Shone complex
- D. All of the options

Answers

ANSWER 1: B. Two-dimensional echocardiography with color Doppler establishes the diagnosis of a subvalvular membrane identified as the cause of left ventricular outflow tract (LVOT) obstruction indicated by a turbulent LVOT flow in the LAX views. The aortic regurgitation is mild to moderate.

In DSAS, the presence of a tissue membrane or fibromuscular ridge in the LVOT can result in variable degrees of outflow tract obstruction and aortic valve leaflet damage, which may cause aortic regurgitation.

ANSWER 2: D. All answers are correct. All mentioned defects can be associated with DSAS.

SUBSEQUENT FINDINGS
See Videos 2-3 and 2-4 and Figures 2-4 and 2-5 of a balloon valvulpoplasty performed on this patient with DSAS.

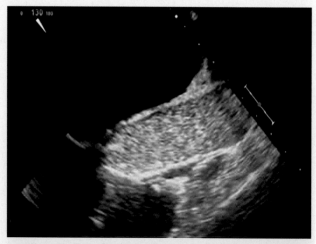

Figure 2-4. Balloon dilatation of the subvalvular membrane.

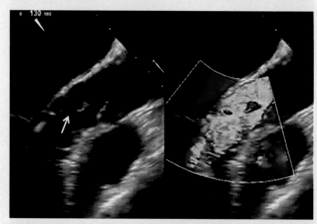

Figure 2-5. TEE 130°, LAX view. After dilatation, parts of the subvalvular membrane (marked with a *white arrow*) can be observed floating in the LVOT.

Suggested Reading

Darcin OT, Yagdi T, Atay Y, et al. Discrete subaortic stenosis: surgical outcomes and follow-up results. *Tex Heart Inst J.* 2003;30: 286–292.

CASE 3

Aortic Stenosis after a Modified Ross Procedure

*T*he patient is a 23-year-old man with a history of aortic stenosis, status post modified Ross procedure at age 9, complicated by complete heart block requiring a pacemaker, which was subsequently converted to a biventricular pacemaker 6 years ago and a battery change 2 years ago. His only complaints have been that he fatigues easily and experiences occasional light-headedness with an increase in activity such as power walking.

Six years ago, a small fistula was found near his left ventricular outflow tract (LVOT). A recent cardiac catheterization demonstrated that his left ventricular outflow fistula had enlarged (Fig. 3-1).

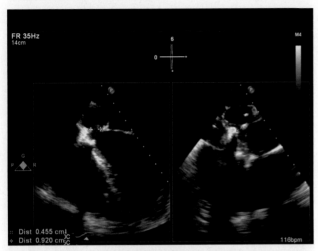

Figure 3-1.

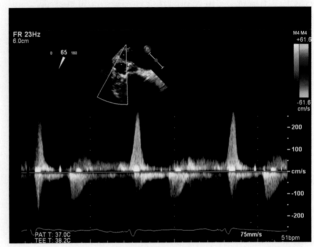

Figure 3-3.

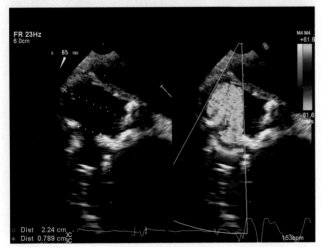

Figure 3-2.

QUESTION 2. The aneurysm does not communicate with another chamber; thus the flow through the aneurysm is going back and forth. In Figure 3-3, the size of the aneurysm is the largest in:

    A. Early systole

    B. Late systole

    C. Early diastole

    D. Late diastole

QUESTION 3. The appropriate management of this intracardiac pseudoaneurysm is:

    A. Medical therapy

    B. Surgery

    C. Transcatheter percutaneous closure

    D. Surgery and transcatheter percutaneous closure

QUESTION 1. The findings of Figures 3-1 and 3-2 are most consistent with:

    A. Intracardiac shunt

    B. Pseudoaneurysm

Answers

ANSWER 1: B. Flow is seen between the aortic out-flow tract and the aortic root. The flow enters a confined space and does not appear to communicate with another intracardiac structure. A computed tomographic angiogram confirmed a 3.5-cm pseudoaneurysm extending from the aortic outflow tract in a posterior direction and an aortic root measuring up to 4.8 cm in maximal diameter.

ANSWER 2: D. Flow across the aneurysm is continuous but the velocity is greatest during early systole – indicating the size of the communication between the aneurysm and LVOT is the smallest at that time.

ANSWER 3: D. The correct management of this patient is closure of the pseudoaneurysm by surgery or transcatheter means. In this case, as shown in Figures 3-4 to 3-6 and Videos 3-1 to 3-3, a percutaneous Amplatzer occluder device was used to close the pseudoaneurysm from LVOT to the posterior left ventricle. Because of the successful procedure, open heart surgery was avoided.

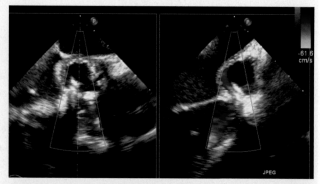

Figure 3-4.

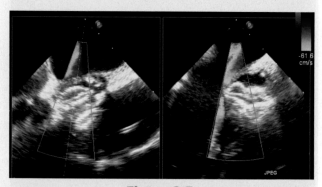

Figure 3-5.

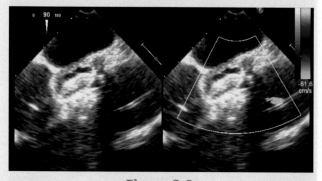

Figure 3-6.

Suggested Readings

Hussain J, Strumpf R, Ghandforoush A, et al. Transcatheter closure of recurrent aortic pseudoaneurysm previously treated by Amplatzer occluder device. *J Vasc Surg*. 2010;52:196–198.

Stasek J, Polansky P, Bis J, et al. The percutaneous closure of a large pseudoaneurysm of the ascending aorta with an atrial septal defect Amplatzer occluder: two-year follow-up. *Can J Cardiol*. 2008;24:e99–e101.

CASE 4

Increasing Shortness of Breath

A 25-year-old medical student had a 6-month history of increasing shortness of breath. Since childhood, he was less physically fit than his classmates, but this was always attributed to his obesity (body mass index of 32). He had no medical history of cardiac disease. A transthoracic echocardiogram was performed, revealing aortic stenosis with a mean gradient of 42 mm Hg and mild aortic regurgitation.

For a more detailed assessment of the aortic valve, a transesophageal echocardiogram (TEE) was performed (Figs. 4-1 to 4-5).

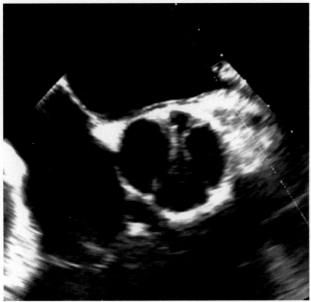

Figure 4-1. 2D TEE: Midesophageal short-axis view (60°) of the aortic valve in diastole.

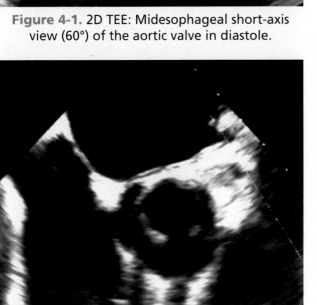

Figure 4-2. 2D TEE: Midesophageal short-axis view (60°) of the aortic valve in systole.

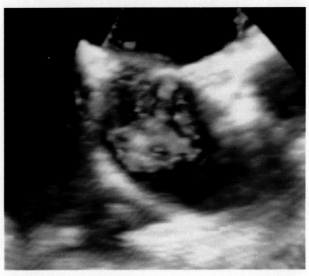

Figure 4-3. 3D TEE: Enface view of the aortic valve in diastole.

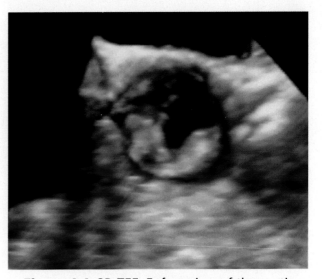

Figure 4-4. 3D TEE: Enface view of the aortic valve in systole.

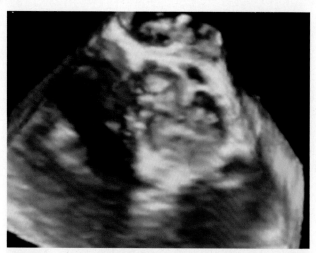

Figure 4-5. 3D TEE: Enface view of the aortic valve.

QUESTION 1. What is his diagnosis?
A. Rheumatic aortic valve disease
B. Bicuspid aortic valve
C. Calcific disease of a trileaflet aortic valve
D. Unicommissural aortic valve
E. Acommissural aortic valve

Answers

ANSWER 1: D. Isolated rheumatic aortic valve stenosis is a rare disease. There is no history of rheumatic fever in the patient's history, and the aortic leaflets are not demonstrating the typical morphology for rheumatic heart disease with cusp thickening and commissural fusion. Therefore, this diagnosis is highly unlikely in this patient.

Bicuspid valves usually have fusion of one of the three commissures (most commonly the left and right), and, echocardiographically, they can be distinguished by the presence of a raphe, creating two functional leaflets orcusps, usually of unequal size.[1,2] Two commissures (or hinge points) are usually present. The aortic valve of our patient demonstrates only one commissure. Additionally, leaflet doming, eccentric closure, and fish mouth orifice during systole represent typical echocardiographic findings of a unicommissural valve.

Calcific disease of a trileaflet aortic valve can be distinguished clinically by age of onset and by characteristic echocardiographic findings. This form of aortic stenosis progresses slowly, and symptoms most frequently occur between ages 70 and 90. Echocardiographically, varying degrees of nodular thickening and calcification of the three leaflets with restricted systolic motion are typically observed, which is not the case in this patient.

A unicuspid aortic valve is a rare condition resulting from abnormal valvulogenesis. The estimated incidence is 0.02% in the adult population.[3]

Two types of unicuspid aortic valves can be differentiated: a unicommissural (more common) and an acommissural unicuspid valve.

The opening of a unicommissural valve is eccentric, and the opening area resembles a "teardrop." An acommissural type of aortic valve has a more centralized, triangular opening area due to an underdevelopment of all three leaflets. The stenosis of an acommissural aortic valve is usually severe and diagnosed in infancy (Figs. 4-6 and 4-7).

Due to the symptoms and relevant aortic stenosis, the patient underwent a Ross operation. Intraoperatively, the diagnosis of a unicuspid aortic valve (unicommissural type) was confirmed.

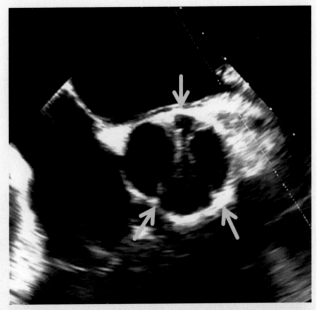

Figure 4-6. 2D TEE: Midesophageal short-axis view (60°) of the aortic valve in diastole. The *yellow arrows* mark what looks like three commissures.

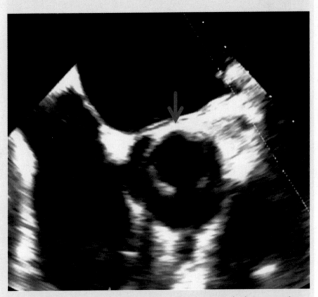

Figure 4-7. 2D TEE: Midesophageal short-axis view (60°) of the aortic valve in systole. The *red arrow* points to the attachment of the leaflet to the aorta, thus indicating that this is a unicommissural aortic valve.

References

1. Roberts WC. Morphologic aspects of cardiac valve dysfunction. *Am Heart J.* 1992;123(6):1610–1632.
2. Roberts WC. The congenitally bicuspid aortic valve. A study of 85 autopsy cases. *Am J Cardiol.* 1970;26(1):72–83.
3. Novaro GM, Mishra M, Griffin BP. Incidence and echocardiographic features of congenital unicuspid aortic valve in adult population. *J Heart Valve Dis.* 2003;12:670–673.

Weakness and Malaise

*T*he patient is a 26-year-old woman who has had weakness and malaise for 1 to 2 months. She has a past history of congenital heart disease, and she had ventricular septal defect (VSD) repair and repair of aortic valve prolapse 8 years ago. See Videos 5-1 to 5-5 and Figures 5-1 to 5-5.

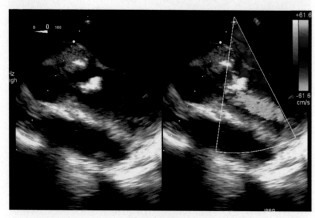

Figure 5-1.

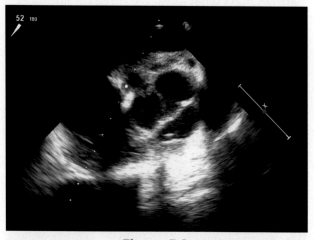

Figure 5-2.

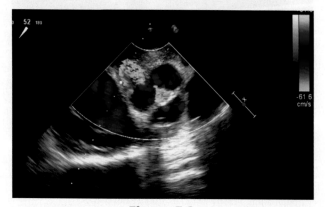

Figure 5-3.

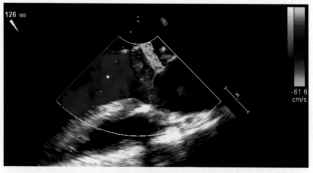

Figure 5-4.

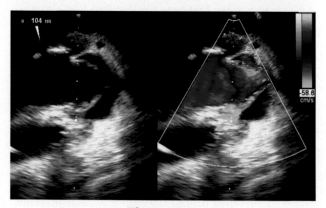

Figure 5-5.

QUESTION 1. In the images, all of the following abnormalities are present *except*:

A. Aortic valve vegetation

B. Aortic root abscess

C. Aortic valve regurgitation

D. Atrial septal defect (ASD)

Answers

ANSWER 1: D. Considering her history of aortic valve surgery and closure of VSD, as well as recent fatigue and weakness, endocarditis should be suspected. The transesophageal echocardiogram images in the figures certainly confirm that there is endocarditis with an aortic root abscess, severe aortic regurgitation, and a large vegetation. A small VSD is seen in the images (not ASD).

Suggested Reading

Leung DY, Cranney GB, Hopkins AP, et al. Role of transesophageal echocardiography in the diagnosis and management of aortic root abscess. *Br Heart J.* 1994;72:175–181.

Dizziness and Near Syncope

A 27-year-old woman complains of dizziness and near syncope. See Figures 6-1 to 6-3.

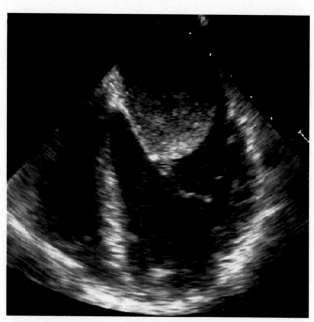

Figure 6-1.

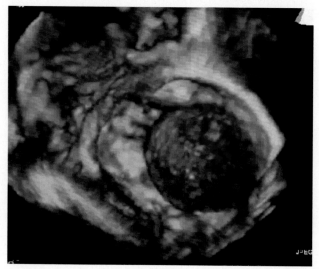

Figure 6-3.

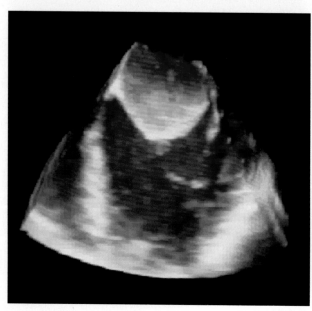

Figure 6-2.

QUESTION 1. Based on the images, what is the most likely diagnosis?

A. Left atrial (LA) myxoma
B. Right atrial thrombus
C. LA thrombus
D. Right atrial sarcoma
E. LA sarcoma

QUESTION 2. What physical findings may you find in this patient?

A. Clubbing and cyanosis
B. A holosystolic murmur over the apex
C. A mid-diastolic rumble
D. A mid-systolic murmur
E. An early diastolic decrescendo murmur

Answers

ANSWER 1: A. The patient has a very large LA mass appearing to be attached to the interatrial septum near the fossa ovalis. There is > 90% likelihood that such a tumor is a myxoma. This tumor is the most common primary cardiac tumor and is seen in > 75% of cases in the left atrium, of which > 90% are attached to the interatrial septum. The tumor is shown in the four-chamber transesophageal echocardiogram (TEE) view with both 2D and 3D as well as in the LA "enface" view (mitral valve below the tumor) using real-time 3D TEE.

ANSWER 2: C. The patient has a very large LA myxoma that appears to obstruct the mitral valve orifice in diastole and thereby may cause symptoms of mitral stenosis, including the mid-diastolic rumble, which, in the case of LA myxoma, may be positional. Such obstruction may also cause presyncope or syncope. Treatment is surgical resection of the tumor upon diagnosis.

Suggested Reading

Neuman Y, Tolstrup K, Siegel RJ, et al. Pseudomyxoma originating from the interatrial septum in a heart transplant patient. *J Am Soc Echo.* 2005;18:771.

Episode of Hemoptysis

A 28-year-old man with a history of childhood surgery for congenital heart disease presents following an episode of hemoptysis. He reports a mild decline in his exercise tolerance during the past month. He had surgery as a child to close "a hole" in his heart but has not seen a physician since that time.

On his physical exam, his blood pressure is 115/75 mm Hg and pulse is 66 beats per minute and regular. His O_2 saturation is 88% on room air. Neck veins are elevated to the angle of the jaw. Carotid pulses are normal. Lungs are clear to auscultation bilaterally. Cardiac exam reveals a normal S1 with a loud P2 component of the second heart sound and a 3/6 holosystolic murmur at the left lower sternal border that is nonradiating. Extremities are warm with no peripheral edema.

Echocardiography is performed to evaluate left ventricular (LV) systolic function (Videos 7-1 and 7-2 and Figs. 7-1 to 7-3).

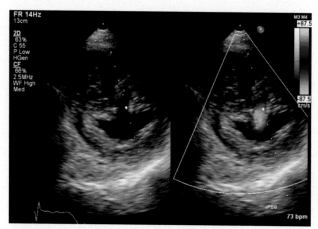

Figure 7-1. Transthoracic echocardiogram (TTE): Short axis view with color Doppler.

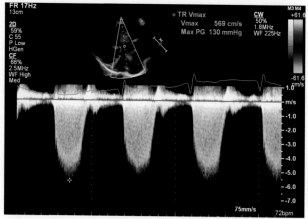

Figure 7-3. TTE RV inflow view with continuous wave (CW) Doppler.

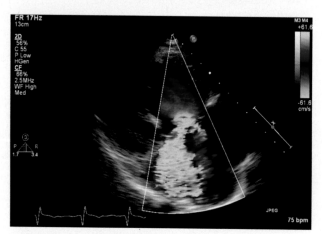

Figure 7-2. TTE RV inflow view with color Doppler.

QUESTION 1. The echocardiogram demonstrates evidence of:

- A. RV pressure overload
- B. RV volume overload
- C. Systemic pulmonary artery pressures
- D. Severe tricuspid regurgitation
- E. All of the options

QUESTION 2. The echocardiogram in Figures 7-1 and 7-4 and Video 7-3 demonstrates evidence of:

- A. A secundum atrial septal defect
- B. An atrioventricular canal defect
- C. A muscular ventricular septal defect (VSD)
- D. A supracristal VSD
- E. A patent ductus arteriosus

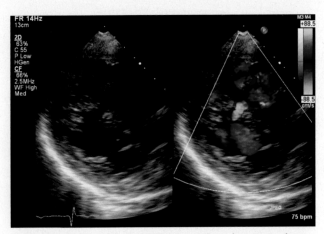

Figure 7-4. TTE, low PLAX with color Doppler.

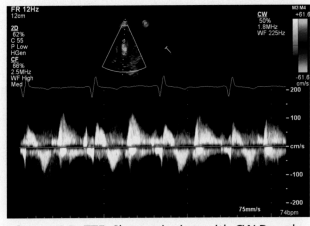

Figure 7-5. TTE: Short axis view with CW Doppler across the VSD.

QUESTION 3. The low systolic flow velocities across the VSD in Figure 7-5 suggests:

    A. The VSD should be closed surgically
    B. The VSD should be closed percutaneously
    C. The VSD is not hemodynamically significant
    D. Eisenmenger syndrome is present
    E. The RV systolic pressure is low

Answers

ANSWER 1: E. All of the options are present. There is evidence of interventricular septal flattening in both systole and diastole, suggestive of RV pressure and volume overload. There is severe pulmonary hypertension with an estimated RV systolic pressure greater than 130 mm Hg. Color Doppler shows severe tricuspid regurgitation with tricuspid valve leaflet malcoaptation.

ANSWER 2: C. There is evidence of a muscular VSD in the distal portion of the interventricular septum. Color flow Doppler demonstrates bidirectional low velocity flow across the VSD.

ANSWER 3: D. This is a nonrestrictive low flow velocity VSD that is seen with Eisenmenger syndrome. Closure of the VSD is contraindicated as it may cause RV failure and death. The most viable treatment option in such a symptomatic patient is either heart–lung transplant or bilateral lung transplant and closure of the VSD.

Suggested Reading

Niwa K, Perloff JK, Kaplan S, et al. Eisenmenger syndrome in adults: ventricular septal defect, truncus arteriosus, univentricular heart. *J Am Coll Cardiol.* 1999;34:223–232.

CASE 8

Atrial Fibrillation

A 30-year-old man with atrial fibrillation presents with the echocardiogram in Video 8-1.

QUESTION 1. What is his underlying congenital abnormality?

    A. Ebstein's anomaly

    B. Tetralogy of Fallot

    C. Atrial septal defect (ASD)

    D. Anomalous pulmonary venous return

QUESTION 2. The right atrial mass (Video 8-1) most likely represents:

    A. Thrombus

    B. Atrial myxoma

    C. Fibroelastoma

    D. None of the options

QUESTION 3. Which mass *cannot* be found in the right atrium (RA)?

    A. Thrombus

    B. Myxoma

    C. Cardiac papillary fibroelastoma

    D. None of the options

Answers

ANSWER 1: A. The RA is enlarged, and the tricuspid annulus is apically displaced into the right ventricle in Ebstein's anomaly.

ANSWER 2: A. Given the patient's enlarged RA from Ebstein's anomaly as well as his history of atrial fibrillation, the most likely etiology of the RA mass is a thrombus; Ebstein's anomaly is not associated with an increased incidence of intracardiac tumors.

ANSWER 3: D. Although a thrombus is by far the most common, any of the options can be found in the RA.

Suggested Reading

Muñoz-Castellanos, Espinola-Zavaleta N, Kuri-Nivón, et al. Ebstein's Anomaly: anatomo-echocardiographic correlation. *Cardiovasc Ultrasound.* 2007;5:43.

Left-Sided Hemiparesis

A 31-year-old woman presented with sudden onset of left-sided hemiparesis. A cardiogenic embolic stroke was suspected and transthoracic echocardiography was performed; Video 9-1 and Figure 9-1 show a transthoracic echo – apical four-chamber view. A transesophageal echo was performed – Videos 9-2 and 9-3 and Figures 9-2 and 9-3.

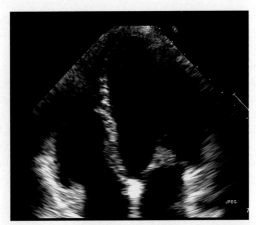

Figure 9-1. Transthoracic echocardiography shows a 0.7 × 0.7 cm mobile mass attached to the anterior mitral leaflet.

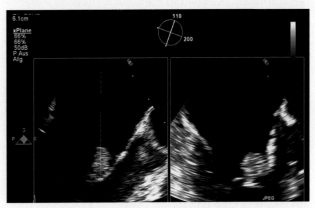

Figure 9-2.

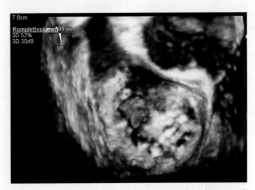

Figure 9-3. 3D transesophageal echocardiogram (TEE) full volume. Enface view of the mitral valve—the mass is attached to the A1 segment of the anterior leaflet.

QUESTION 1. How would you proceed to confirm a diagnosis?

A. Perform laboratory tests
B. Perform a transesophageal echocardiogram
C. Perform a magnetic resonance imaging
D. Start anticoagulation therapy immediately
E. Send the patient to surgery

QUESTION 2. The structure attached to the A1 segment of the anterior leaflet of the mitral valve is most likely:

A. An organized mobile thrombus
B. Nonbacterial thrombotic endocarditis
C. A pedunculated myxoma
D. Libman-Sacks endocarditis
E. A cardiac papillary fibroelastoma (CPF)

Answers

ANSWER 1: A. Laboratarory data should be collected to exclude infective endocarditis or malignant diseases causing nonbacterial thrombotic endocarditis. A systemic lupus erythematosus should be excluded as well (Libman-Sacks endocarditis).

Anticoagulation therapy is an option to prevent possible recurrent embolism due to superimposed thrombus formation attached to the cardiac mass.

A TEE should be performed to differentiate among intracardiac tumors, particularly among CPF, myxoma, and vegetation of endocarditis.

ANSWER 2: E. A thrombotic mass usually shows an echolucent area in the middle due to clot lysis. A thrombus appears multilayered with irregular or lobulated borders. In > 90% of cases, a thrombus is located in the left atrial appendage.

A myxoma is usually larger and more heterogeneous compared to CPF, and in the majority of cases, myxomas are located in the left atrium.

Vegetations are usually irregular in shape and echogenic. Vegetations show high-frequency movements independent of intracardiac structures.

CPF is a rare benign tumor that attaches to the endocardial surface, most often on cardiac valves. A CPF is most often solitary and more frequently located on the aortic valve (44%) than on the mitral valve (35%).[1-3]

Echocardiographic findings for CPF include a round, oval, or irregular appearant homogeneous tumor mass with well-defined borders. Most CPFs are small (90% < 20 mm), and approximately 50% have small stems and are highly mobile. The moving behavior on echocardiography is similar to the flexion–extension movement of a finger.[2,4]

The 2D and 3D echo findings are indicative of CPF in this case. The treatment for CPF is excision of the tumor.

The patient was sent for surgery, and the histopathologic findings confirmed the diagnosis of a CPF.

References

1. Gowda RM, Khan IA, Nair CK, et al. Cardiac papillary fibroelastoma: a comprehensive analysis of 725 cases. *Am Heart J.* 1992;146:157–162.
2. Sun JP, Asher CR, Yang XS, et al. Clinical and echocardiographic characteristics of papillary fibroelastoma: a retrospective and prospective study in 162 patients. *Circulation.* 2001;103:2687–2693.
3. Eslami-Varzaneh F, Brun EA, Sears-Rogan P. An unusual case of multiple papillary fibroelastoma, review of literature. *Cardiovasc Pathol.* 2003;12:170–173.
4. Baba Y, Tsuboi Y, Sakiyama K, et al. Cardiac papillary fibroelastoma as a cause of recurrent strokes: the diagnostic value of serial transesophageal echocardiography. *Cerebrovasc Dis.* 2002;14:256–259.

CASE 10

Dyspnea on Exertion

A 32-year-old man complains of dyspnea on exertion. He also has acroparathesias, anhidrosis, and normal blood pressure. His father has renal disease. His electrocardiogram (Fig. 10-1) and echocardiogram (Videos 10-1 to 10-3 and Figs. 10-2 and 10-3) are shown.

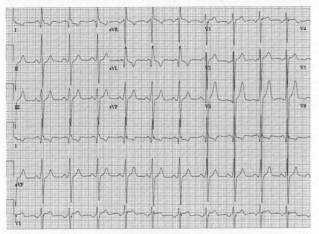

Figure 10-1.

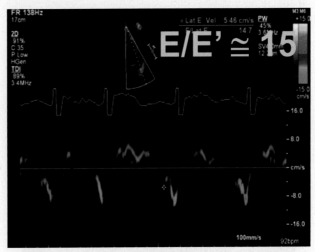

Figure 10-3.

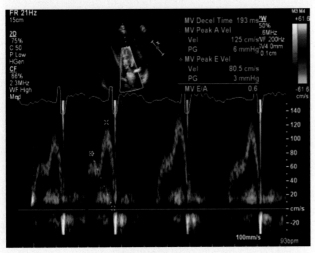

Figure 10-2.

QUESTION 1. The most likely diagnosis is:

A. Amyloid

B. Sarcoid

C. Hypertensive heart disease

D. Fabry disease

Answers

ANSWER 1: D. The presence of acroparesthesias, anhidrosis, and paternal history of renal disease all suggest Fabry disease, which is an X-linked disorder that is associated with renal dysfunction.

The echocardiographic findings include left ventricular hypertrophy (LVH) and a bright subendocardial layer as shown in Video 10-4 and Figures 10-4 and 10-5 in our patient and a published case.

The LVH and right ventricular hypertrophy in Fabry disease are due to the accumulation of glycosphingolipids (SM) as shown in Figure 10-5.

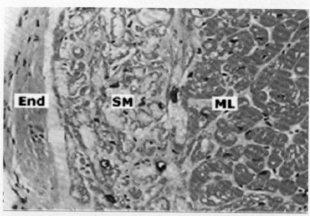

Figure 10-5. Reprinted from Pieroni M, Chimenti C, De Cobelli F, et al. Fabry's disease cardiomyopathy: echocardiographic detection of endomyocardial glycosphingolipid compartmentalization. *J AM Coll Cardiol.* 2006;47:1663–1671, with permission from Elsevier.

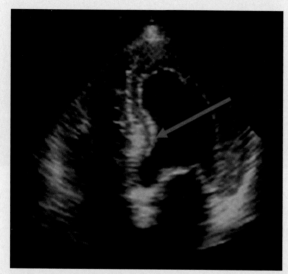

Figure 10-4. Reprinted from Pieroni M, Chimenti C, De Cobelli F, et al. Fabry's disease cardiomyopathy: echocardiographic detection of endomyocardial glycosphingolipid compartmentalization. *J AM Coll Cardiol.* 2006;47:1663–1671, with permission from Elsevier.

Suggested Reading

Pieroni M, Chimenti C, De Cobelli F, et al. Fabry's disease cardiomyopathy: echocardiographic detection of endomyocardial glycosphingolipid compartmentalization. *J Am Coll Cardiol.* 2006; 47:1663–1671.

CASE 11

Marfan Syndrome

A 32-year-old man with Marfan syndrome has a screening transthoracic echocardiogram performed (Fig. 11-1).

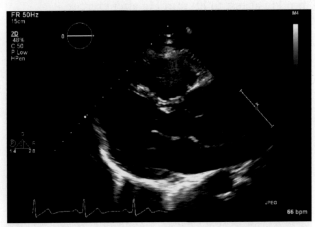

Figure 11-1.

QUESTION 1. At what diameter should a patient with Marfan syndrome be considered for surgical repair of an ascending aortic aneurysm?

- A. Greater than 5 cm
- B. Greater than 4 cm and contemplating pregnancy
- C. When the maximum aortic root area (cm²) per height in meters is < 10
- D. Answers A and B are correct
- E. All of the options

Answers

ANSWER 1: D. Indications for the repair of the ascending aorta or root in Marfan syndrome:
- Greater than 5 cm
- Less than 5 cm and:
  - Growth > 0.5 cm per year
  - Family history of dissection < 5 cm
  - Concomitant significant aortic insufficiency
- Greater than 4 cm and contemplating pregnancy
- When the maximum aortic root area (cm²) per height in meters is > 10

Suggested Reading

Hiratzka LF, Bakris GL, Beckman JA, et al. Guidelines for the diagnosis and management of patients with thoracic aortic disease: a report of the American College of Cardiology Foundation/American Heart Association Task Force on Practice Guidelines, American Association for Thoracic Surgery, American College of Radiology, American Stroke Association, Society of Cardiovascular Anesthesiologists, Society for Cardiovascular Angiography and Interventions, Society of Interventional Radiology, Society of Thoracic Surgeons, and Society for Vascular Medicine. *J Am Coll Cardiol.* 2010;55:e27–e129.

CASE 12

Shortness of Breath and Dyspnea on Exertion

A 33-year-old man from India complains of shortness of breath and dyspnea on exertion (DOE) walking one to two blocks.

On an exercise test, he exercised for 8 minutes 41 seconds, reaching a heart rate of 181 beats per minute. His pulmonary artery pressure increased from 48 mm Hg at rest to 89 mm Hg after exercise.

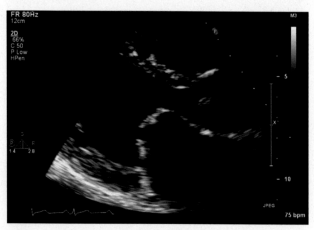

Figure 12-1.

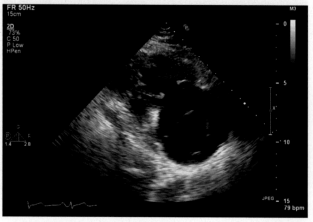

Figure 12-3.

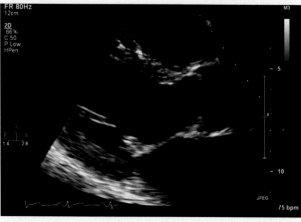

Figure 12-2.

QUESTION 1. Figures 12-1 to 12-3 are consistent with:

A. Rheumatic mitral valve disease
B. Rheumatic valvular disease of the aortic valve
C. Rheumatic valvular disease of mitral, aortic, and tricuspid valves
D. Rheumatic mitral and aortic valve disease
E. Degenerative valvular disease

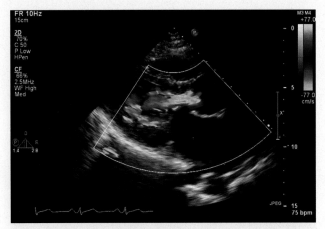

Figure 12-4.

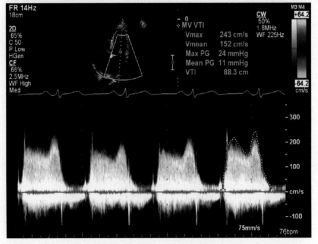

Figure 12-5.

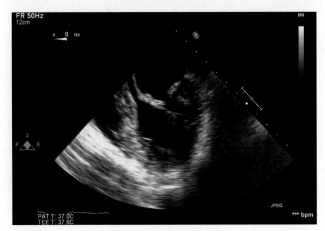

Figure 12-6.

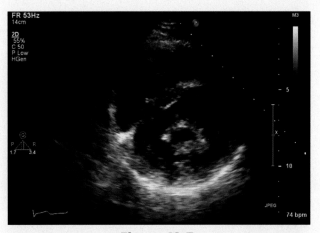

Figure 12-7.

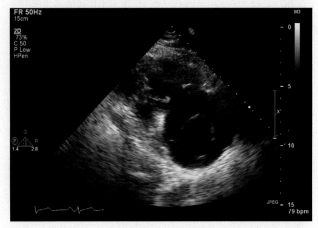

Figure 12-8.

QUESTION 3. Based on the echocardiogram images in Figures 12-6 and 12-7, this patient is not a candidate for percutaneous mitral valvuloplasty because:

A. He does not have isolated severe MS

B. He has extensive valvular and subvalvular calcifications

C. He has at least moderate mitral regurgitation (MR)

D. All of the options are true

E. None of the options are true

QUESTION 4. Based on the echocardiogram image in Figure 12-8, the round structure in the middle of the right atrium is:

A. An artifact

B. A prominent Eustachian valve

C. Chiari network

D. An interatrial septal aneurysm

E. A tumor

QUESTION 2. Based on the echo images in Figures 12-4 and 12-5, the patient has the following:

A. No significant mitral stenosis (MS); significant aortic regurgitation (AR)

B. Significant MS and AR

C. No significant AR; significant MS

D. No significant valvular disease

Answers

ANSWER 1: C. All three valves demonstrate thickening of the leaflet tips with diastolic doming of the mitral and tricuspid valves and systolic doming of the aortic valve. Typically, the mitral valve is most commonly affected followed by the aortic valve, and when the aortic valve is affected, the mitral valve is almost invariably affected. It is much more uncommon to have the tricuspid valve involved.

ANSWER 2: B. Figure 12-4 demonstrates a diastolic frame in the parasternal long-axis view, showing severe aortic valve regurgitation: AR vena contracta is greater than 0.6 cm and takes up almost the whole outflow tract. A high velocity jet is seen within the left ventricle, suggesting MS. The significance of the MS is shown in Figure 12-5 using continuous wave across the mitral valve in the apical four-chamber view. The mean diastolic pressure gradient of 11 mm Hg is consistent with severe MS.

ANSWER 3: E. While extensive calcification of the mitral valve and subvalvular apparatus would increase the Wilkins score and make percutaneous balloon valvuloplasty less likely to be successful (Wilkins score ≥ 8), there is no evidence of significant calcifications of this valve or subvalvular apparatus. Also, although moderate to greater degree of MR is a contraindication to balloon valvuloplasty, severe aortic valve regurgitation is not.

ANSWER 4: D. The transthoracic image in Figure 12-8 demonstrates an enface view of an interatrial septal aneurysm from a right ventricular inflow perspective.

In this patient with high left atrial pressure, this is also demonstrated by the left-to-right bowing of the aneurysm on the transesophageal images shown in Figure 12-9.

Table 12-1 summarizes classification of severity of MS and AR by echocardiography.

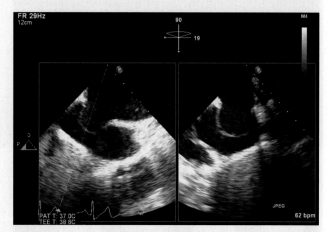

Figure 12-9.

Answers

TABLE 12-1. Classification of Severity of MS and AR by Echocardiography

	Mitral Stenosis		
	Mild	Moderate	Severe
Mean gradient (mm Hg)	Less than 5	5–10	Greater than 10
Pulmonary artery systolic pressure (mm Hg)	Less than 30	30–50	Greater than 50
Valve area (cm²)	Greater than 1.5	1.0–1.5	Less than 1.0

	Aortic Regurgitation		
	Mild	Moderate	Severe
Qualitative			
Angiographic grade	1+	2+	3–4+
Color Doppler jet width	Central jet, width less than 25% of LVOT	Greater than mild but no signs of severe AR	Central jet, width greater than 65% LVOT
Doppler vena contracta width (cm)	Less than 0.3	0.3–0.6	Greater than 0.6

Reprinted from Bonow RO, Carabello BA, Nishimura RA, et al. 2008 focused update incorporated into the ACC/AHA 2006 guidelines for the management of patients with valvular heart disease: a report of the American College of Cardiology/American Heart Association Task Force on Practice Guidelines (Writing Committee to revise the 1998 guidelines for the management of patients with valvular heart disease). Endorsed by the Society of Cardiovascular Anesthesiologists, Society for Cardiovascular Angiography and Interventions, and Society of Thoracic Surgeons. *J Am Coll Cardiol*. 2008;52(13):e1–e142.

CASE 13

AIDS and *Pneumocystis* Pneumonia

A 34-year-old woman with AIDS and a history of *Pneumocystis* pneumonia presents with shortness of breath and hemoptysis. She is hypoxic and hypotensive on presentation. See Figures 13-1 and 13-2.

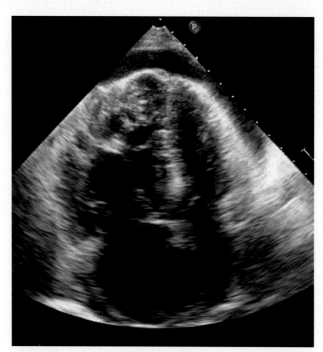

Figure 13-1.

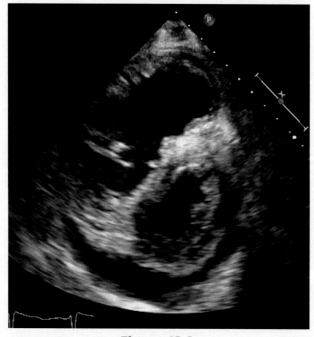

Figure 13-2.

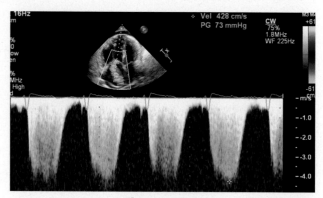

Figure 13-3.

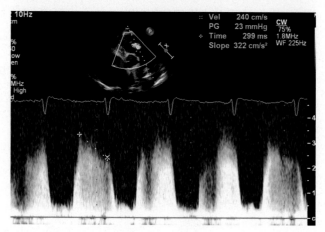

Figure 13-4.

QUESTION 1. The following is true *except*:

A. The patient has marked right ventricular (RV) dilatation with hypertrophy

B. The patient has evidence of RV pressure overload

C. The patient has a moderate pericardial effusion

D. All are correct

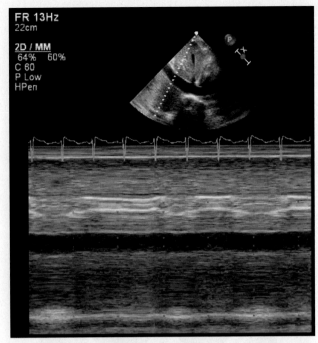

Figure 13-5.

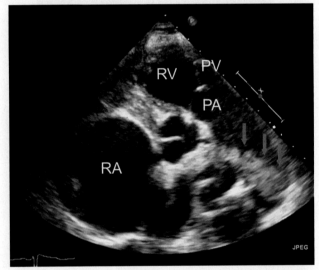

Figure 13-6.

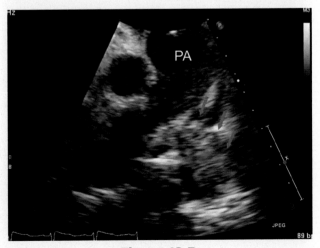

Figure 13-7.

QUESTION 2. Based on the echocardiogram images in Figures 13-3 to 13-5, the following statement is true about the patient's pulmonary hypertension:

    A. The pulmonary artery (PA) systolic pressure is severely elevated, the PA diastolic pressure is mildly elevated, and right atrial (RA) pressure is normal

    B. The PA systolic pressure is moderately elevated, the PA diastolic pressure is moderately elevated, and RA pressure is elevated

    C. The PA systolic pressure is severely elevated, the PA diastolic pressure is severely elevated, and RA pressure is elevated

    D. The PA systolic pressure is moderately elevated, the PA diastolic pressure is severely elevated, and RA pressure is elevated

QUESTION 3. All of the following are possible causes of this patient's severe pulmonary hypertension *except*:

    A. A large atrial septal defect (ASD)

    B. Long-standing lung disease with recurrent pneumonias

    C. Chronic or acute on chronic thromboembolic disease

    D. Acute pulmonary embolus

QUESTION 4. The arrows in Figures 13-6 and 13-7 point to:

    A. A thrombus in a patent ductus arteriosus

    B. A thrombus in the proximal left PA

    C. A thrombus in the proximal right PA

Answers

ANSWER 1: D. The images demonstrate a markedly enlarged right ventricle with severe RV hypertrophy. There is flattening of the interventricular septum in systole consistent with right ventricular (RV) pressure overload. With RV volume overload, the septum would be flattened only in diastole. The left ventricular (LV) cavity is small, and there is a moderate pericardial effusion.

ANSWER 2: C. The patient has severe tricuspid regurgitation (TR) with an RV-to-RA pressure gradient of 73 mm Hg based on the continuous wave of the TR signal. The inferior vena cava is non-to-minimally collapsing, consistent with an estimated RA pressure of 15 mm Hg. Therefore, the estimated PA systolic pressure is severely elevated at 88 mm Hg. The PA diastolic pressure is calculated as 4 v^2 of the end-diastolic pulmonary regurgitation (PR) velocity plus the central venous pressure (CVP), that is 23 mm Hg plus 15 mm Hg = 38 mm Hg—also severely elevated. The mean PA pressure can be calculated as the pressure gradient of the early diastolic PR flow plus the CVP, here an estimated 36 mm Hg plus 15 mm Hg = 51 mm Hg—also severely elevated.

ANSWER 3: D. Large ASDs with long-standing right-to-left shunts may cause severe pulmonary hypertension with resultant dilatation of the RV and development of RV hypertrophy. Therefore, a study should be performed to rule out an ASD. Chronic lung disease and chronic pulmonary embolism likewise can cause severe pulmonary hypertension with affection of the right heart. An acute pulmonary embolism alone would potentially cause an acute dilatation of the RV, but there would be no hypertrophy. Also, most large acute pulmonary emboli cause pulmonary hypertension only in the moderate range.

ANSWER 4: B. The patient had a history of chronic thrombotic disease and pulmonary hypertension but presented acutely with a large occlusive thrombus in the proximal left PA, causing her deterioration.

The echocardiogram findings are confirmed by the computed tomography scan. Arrows point to thrombus (Fig. 13-8).

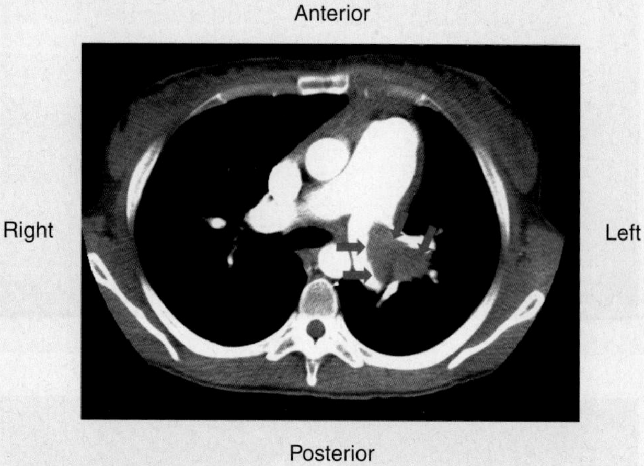

Figure 13-8. Computed tomography scan of occlusive thrombus in left PA.

Suggested Reading

Miniati M, Monti S, Pratali L, et al. Value of transthoracic echocardiography in the diagnosis of pulmonary embolism: results of a prospective study in unselected patients. *Am J Med.* 2001;110:528–535.

Congenital Heart Disease

A 34-year-old woman is referred for evaluation for congenital heart disease.

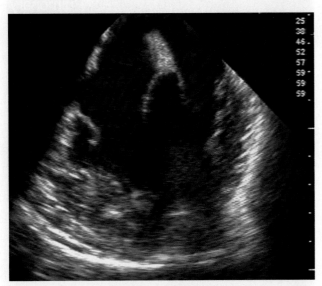

Figure 14-1A.

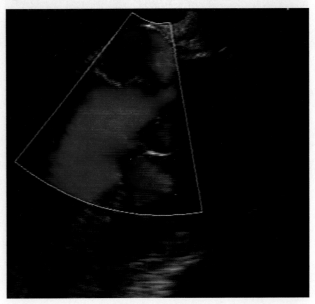

Figure 14-1C.

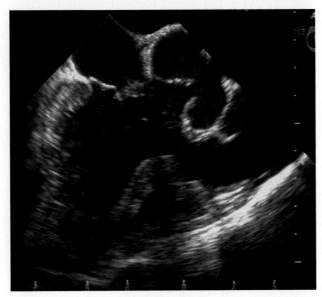

Figure 14-1B.

QUESTION 1. Based on the image provided (Fig. 14-1), the patient can be diagnosed with:

    A. Hypoplastic left heart and tricuspid atresia
    B. Transposition of the great arteries
    C. Double inlet left ventricle
    D. An ASD and a ventricular septal defect (VSD)
    E. All of the options

Answers

ANSWER 1: E. The images show a double inlet left ventricle with a rudimentary right ventricle with left-to-right blood flow through a VSD (Fig. 14-2). An ASD is visualized on Figure 14-2A.

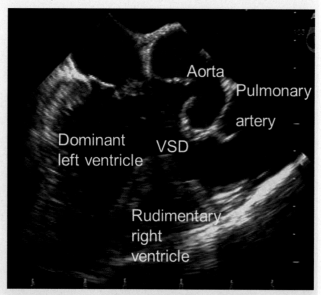

Figure 14-2B.

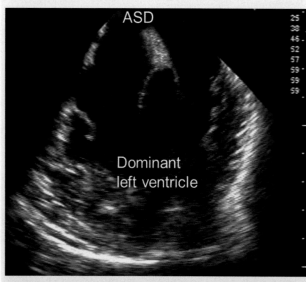

Figure 14-2A.

Suggested Reading

Ammash NM, Warnes CA. Survival into adulthood of patients with unoperated single ventricle. *Am J Cardiol.* 1996;77:542–544.

CASE 15

Family History of Sudden Cardiac Death

A 35-year-old woman with a family history of sudden cardiac death comes for cardiac evaluation (Videos 15-1 to 15-5 and Figs. 15-1 to 15-4).

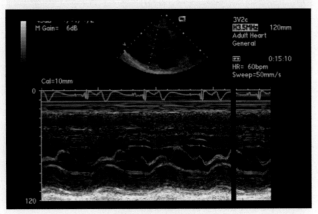

Figure 15-1.

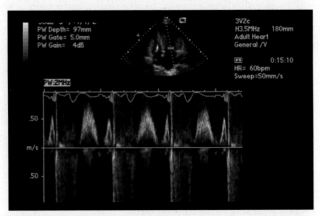

Figure 15-2. Pulse and continuous wave Doppler, mitral inflow.

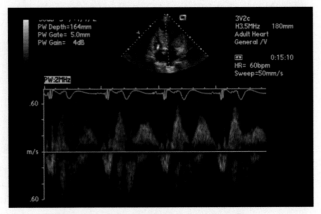

Figure 15-3. Pulmonary vein flow.

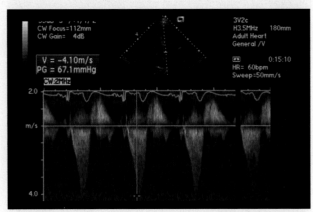

Figure 15-4. LVOT peak PGr = 67.1 mm Hg.

QUESTION 1. This echocardiogram demonstrates findings most consistent with:

A. Hypertrophic cardiomyopathy (HCM)
B. Pompe disease
C. Hypertensive cardiomyopathy
D. Discrete membranous subaortic stenosis

QUESTION 2. Echocardiogram findings include which of the following (select all that apply)?

A. Systolic anterior motion of the mitral valve (SAM)
B. Cavity obliteration
C. Bright subendocardial stripe
D. Color Doppler demonstrating a concomitant mitral regurgitation (MR) and increased left ventricular outflow tract (LVOT) velocities
E. Echogenic structure consistent with an implantable defibrillator

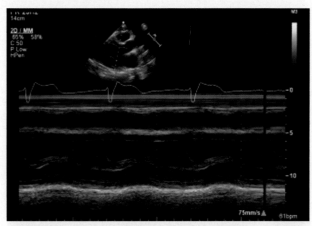

Figure 15-5.

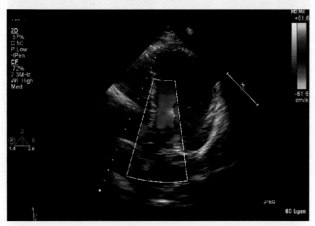

Figure 15-6.

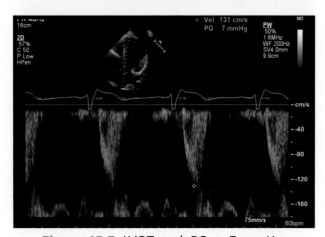

Figure 15-7. LVOT peak PGr = 7 mm Hg.

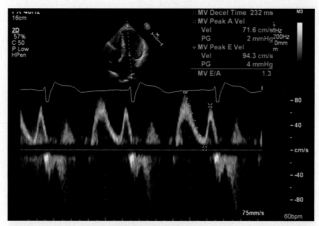

Figure 15-8.

QUESTION 3. The Doppler findings show (select all that apply):

  A. Normal mitral inflow pattern and normal pulmonary vein pattern

  B. Pseudonormal mitral inflow pattern and systolic flow reversal in the pulmonary vein consistent with severe MR

  C. An abnormally increased LVOT gradient

  D. A continuous wave (CW) gradient showing late systolic MR

QUESTION 4. The echocardiographic images (Videos 15-6 to 15-12 and Figs. 15-5 to 15-10) demonstrate which of the following?

  A. Resolution of the SAM

  B. Marked reduction in MR

  C. Marked reduction in LVOT gradient

  D. All of the options

  E. None of the options

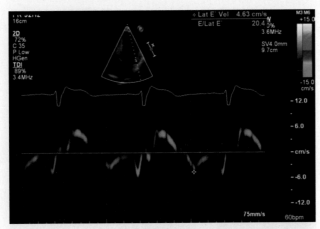

Figure 15-9.

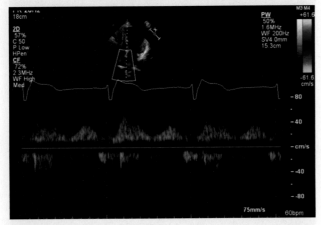

Figure 15-10.

QUESTION 5. The pulse and tissue Doppler indicate (select all that apply):

A. Normal hemodynamics and normalization of the mitral inflow abnormalities

B. Resolution of the LVOT gradient

C. Persistence of pseudonormal mitral inflow pattern

D. Resolution of the pulmonary systolic reversal flow

E. Brain natriuretic peptide (BNP) level is likely to be elevated

QUESTION 6. The change in the echocardiogram Doppler findings is most likely due to:

A. Aggressive therapy with a beta-blocker and disopyramide

B. Surgical myectomy

C. Alcohol septal ablation

D. Rehydration of hypovolemic patient

Answers

ANSWER 1: A. The patient has asymmetric septal hypertrophy, SAM, and LVOT gradient.

ANSWER 2: A, B, D, E. A bright subendocardial stripe, which is not present, is associated with Fabry disease. A defibrillator was placed, as this patient had multiple risk factors for sudden cardiac death including family history, episodes of syncope, and ventricular tachycardia on a Holter monitor.

ANSWER 3: B, C. Of note in patients with HCM and significant increase in wall thickness, a normal mitral inflow is almost always indicative of diastolic dysfunction and elevated filling pressures. The CW gradient in Figure 15-11 has a characteristic dagger shape and late systolic peak of the LVOT velocities seen in HCM patients with LVOT gradients.

ANSWER 4: D. The patient has resolution of the SAM, marked reduction in MR, and marked reduction in LVOT gradient.

ANSWER 5: B, C, D, E. There is resolution of the LVOT gradient and resolution of the pulmonary vein systolic flow reversal flow but a pseudonormal mitral inflow pattern and markedly elevated E/E' (ratio of E wave left ventricular [LV] filling to the myocardial E' wave in diastole), which is likely to be consistent with an elevated BNP. In HCM, in spite of the gradient-reducing therapies, patients still have significant left ventricular hypertrophy (LVH) as well as associated myocardial fibrosis and diastolic dysfunction (the A wave duration on the pulmonary venous flow is increased, the E/E' is elevated, and in a patient with LVH, the expected mitral inflow pattern is E/A [ratio of E wave to A wave velocities during cardiac filling] reversal).

ANSWER 6: B. The answer is surgical myectomy as her basal septum appears considerably thinner, and on short-axis 2D views, a groove at the site of myectomy is apparent (Fig. 15-12, *arrow*).

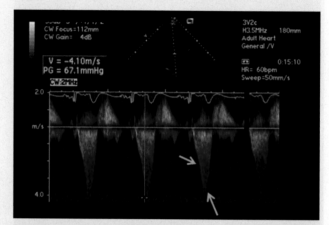

Figure 15-11.

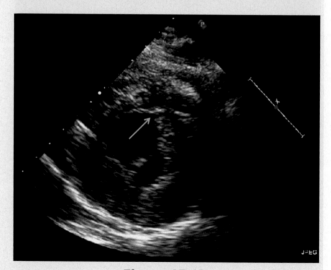

Figure 15-12.

Suggested Reading

Schönbeck MH, Brunner-La Rocca HP, Vogt PR, et al. Long-term follow up in hypertrophic obstructive cardiomyopathy after septal myectomy. *Ann Thorac Surg.* 1998;65:1207–1214.

End-stage Renal Disease on Hemodialysis

*T*he patient is a 35-year-old woman who has a significant past medical history of end-stage renal disease on hemodialysis through a PermCath (Covidien, Mansfield, Massachusetts) and was admitted in septic shock. The patient was transferred to the intensive care unit and now has multiple positive blood cultures.

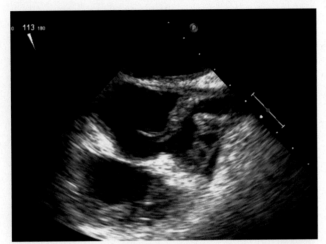

Figure 16-1.

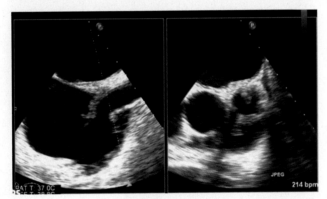

Figure 16-2.

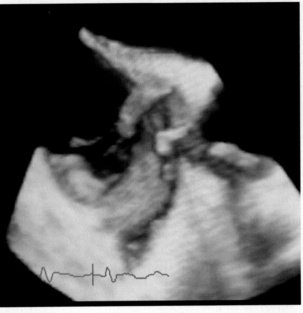

Figure 16-3.

QUESTION 1. Figures 16-1 to 16-3 show:

  A. A vegetation attached to the left atrial (LA) and left pulmonary vein connection
  B. A thrombus attached to the anterior right atrial (RA) to superior vena cava (SVC) connection
  C. A vegetation attached to the posterior RA to SVC connection
  D. A thrombus attached to the LA body to appendage connection

Answers

ANSWER 1: C. Considering the positive culture, the mobile structure is likely infected, that is, a vegetation. Its location is the posterior RA and SVC connection area. A 3D transesophageal echocardiogram provides rotational views of the shape and motion of the vegetation.

Suggested Reading

Sandroni S, McGill R, Brouwer D. Hemodialysis catheter-associated endocarditis: clinical features, risks, and costs. *Semin Dial.* 2003;16:263–265.

CASE 17

Flu with Recent Onset of Congestive Heart Failure

*T*he patient is a 36-year-old woman with a history of the flu 6 weeks prior to admission and onset of congestive heart failure in the last 10 days. See Figures 17-1 and 17-2 and Videos 17-1 and 17-2.

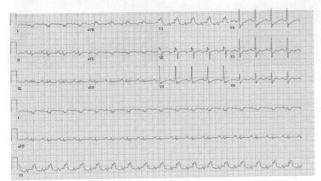

Figure 17-1. Twelve-lead ECG.

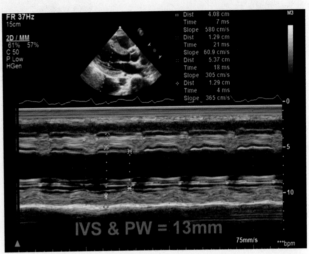

Figure 17-2. There was an increase in the LV wall from 10 mm to 13 mm in 7 days.

QUESTION 1. All of the following are true *except*:

A. The patient has severe left ventricular (LV) dysfunction

B. There is LV mass–electrocardiogram (ECG) voltage discordance

C. The increase in LV wall thickness is best explained by amyloid

D. The increase in LV wall thickness is best explained by myocarditis

Answers

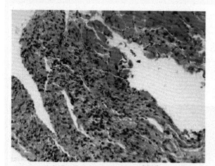 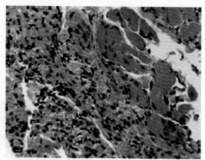 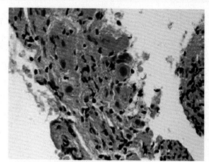

A1-1: myocarditis   A1-2: inflammatory cells   A1-3: myofiber degeneration

Figure 17-3.

ANSWER 1: C. This patient was found to have acute fulminant myocarditis as shown in the histology Figure 17-3 (A1-1; A1-2; A1-3).

Echocardiogram features of acute fulminant myocarditis include the following:

LV with or without right ventricular (RV) systolic dysfunction, which may be global or segmental. There is often an acute increase in LV wall thickness that can also be seen in acute cardiac transplant rejection.

There is a variable natural history. The differential diagnosis for ECG LV voltage–echo mass discordance includes amyloidosis, but in the acute setting it suggests myocarditis.

Fatigue, Weight Loss, and Anorexia

*T*he patient is a 37-year-old man with fatigue, a 20-lb weight loss, and worsening anorexia over the past 6 months.

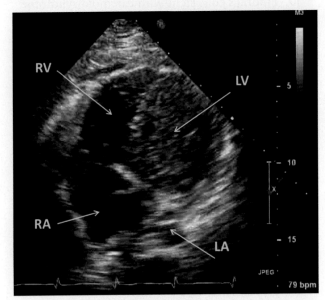

Figure 18-1.

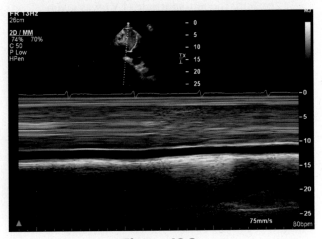

Figure 18-2.

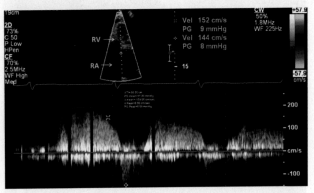

Figure 18-3.

QUESTION 1. A saline contrast bubble study was ordered to evaluate for a patent foramen ovale (PFO). Saline contrast was injected into the right arm.

In Figure 18-1 and Video 18-1, what do you see?

A. A right-to-left shunt consistent with a PFO

B. A ventricular septal defect

C. An atrial septal defect

D. Saline contrast entering the left atrium before the right atrium

QUESTION 2. Based on the M-mode inferior vena cava (IVC) findings (Fig. 18-2), the right atrial pressure is:

A. Normal

B. Elevated

C. Low

QUESTION 3. The spectral Doppler (Fig. 18-3) shows:

A. An increased diastolic gradient across the tricuspid valve

B. Tricuspid regurgitation

C. Pulmonic stenosis

D. Findings consistent with carcinoid syndrome

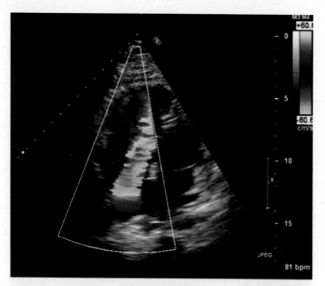

Figure 18-4.

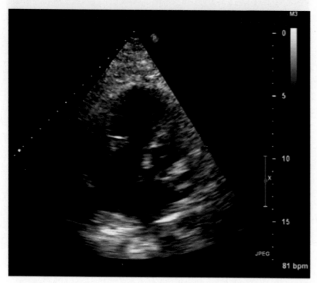

Figure 18-5.

QUESTION 4. In Figure 18-4 and Video 18-2, the apical four-chamber color Doppler views demonstrate:

A. Tricuspid stenosis

B. Diastolic flow convergence across the right ventricular (RV) inflow tract

C. Tricuspid regurgitation

D. Findings consistent with carcinoid syndrome

QUESTION 5. In Figure 18-5 and Video 18-3, the apical four-chamber views demonstrate:

A. Tricuspid stenosis

B. Findings consistent with carcinoid syndrome

C. A Gerbode defect

D. A right atrial mass

QUESTION 6. What is the mechanism responsible for the saline contrast bubbles entering the left atrium before the right atrium?

A. There is an arteriovenous fistula

B. This patient has corrected transposition of the great vessels

C. An echocardiogram contrast agent used to opacify the left ventricle (LV) was given instead of saline

D. There is a right atrial mass obstructing the superior vena cava

Answers

ANSWER 1: D. Saline contrast enters the left atrium before saline contrast is seen in the right atrium.

ANSWER 2: B. Right atrial pressure is elevated, as there is no inspiratory decrease in IVC size.

ANSWER 3: A. The spectral Doppler shows an increased diastolic gradient across the tricuspid valve.

ANSWER 4: B. The apical four-chamber color Doppler views demonstrate diastolic flow convergence across the RV inflow tract.

ANSWER 5: D. The apical four-chamber views demonstrate a right atrial mass.

ANSWER 6: D. There is a right atrial mass obstructing the superior vena cava.

This led to collaterals from the azygous and hemiazygos vein to the left upper pulmonary vein as shown on the computed tomography scans in Figures 18-6 and 18-7 (Reprinted from Beigel R, Thomson LEJ, Siegel RJ. An unusual case of saline contrast injected in the anterior cubital vein appearing in the left heart prior to the right heart. *J Am Coll Cardiol*. In Press, with permission from Elsevier.).

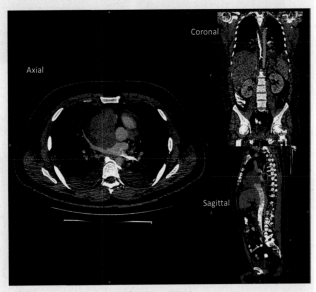

Figure 18-6.

Answers

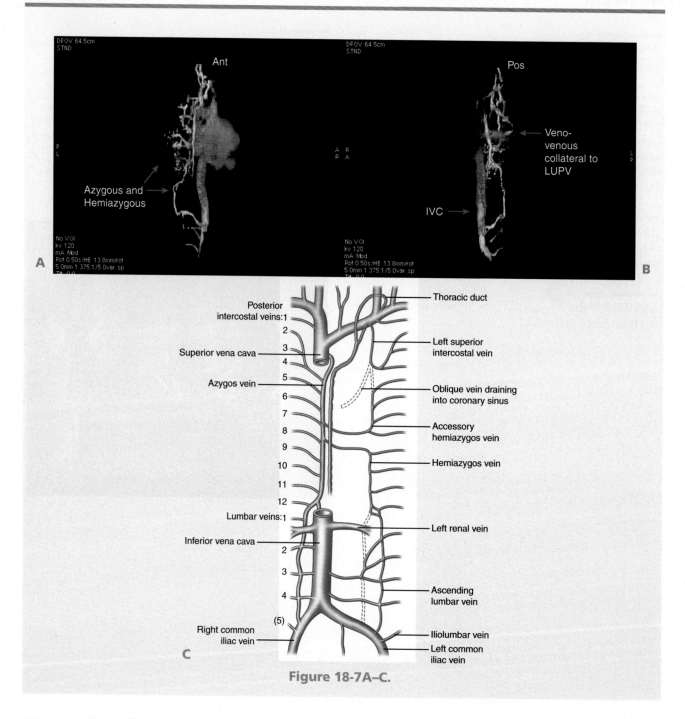

Figure 18-7A–C.

Suggested Reading

Grayet D, Ghaye B, Szapiro D, et al. Systemic-to-pulmonary venous shunt in superior vena cava obstruction revealed on dynamic helical CT. *AJR Am J Roentgenol.* 2001;176:211–213.

CASE 19

Syncope

A 3D transesophageal echocardiogram (TEE) (Video 19-1) and M-mode (Fig. 19-1) are shown for a 37-year-old woman with syncope.

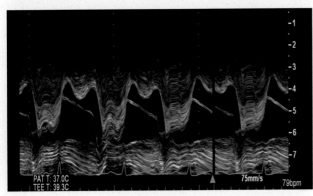

Figure 19-1.

QUESTION 1. The abnormality shown is:

A. Aortic stenosis
B. Left atrial myxoma
C. Infective endocarditis
D. Mitral valve prolapse
E. None of the options

Answers

ANSWER 1: B. The 3D TEE video shows the mitral valve from the left ventricular perspective. The myxoma enters the left ventricle during diastole.

In the M-mode image (Fig. 19-2), the mitral valve (*A*) is seen (*arrow*), and the myxoma (*B*) prolapses into the mitral orifice with each diastole.

Additional 2D TEE images clearly show the myxoma and Doppler diastolic mitral gradient (Videos 19-2 to 19-6 and Fig. 19-3).

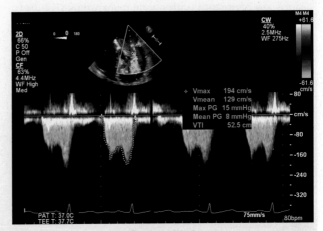

Figure 19-3.

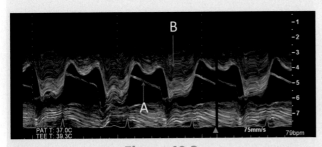

Figure 19-2.

Suggested Reading

Tolstrup K, Shiota T, Gurudevan S, et al. Left atrial myxomas: correlation of two-dimensional and live three-dimensional transesophageal echocardiography with the clinical and pathologic findings. *J Am Soc Echocardiogr.* 2011;24:618–624.

CASE 20

Lip and Skin Lesions with the Appearance of Blebs/Papules

A 38-year-old healthy woman developed lip and skin lesions with the appearance of blebs/papules 2 months ago.

She had swelling of her legs, progressive dyspnea on exertion, fatigue for 2 weeks, and paroxysmal nocturnal dyspnea for 4 days.

QUESTION 1. The findings in Videos 20-1 to 20-4 are most consistent with:

    A. Ischemic cardiomyopathy

    B. Cardiomyopathy due to valvular disease

    C. Acute perimyocarditis

    D. Peripartum cardiomyopathy

    E. Idiopathic cardiomyopathy

QUESTION 2. Based on the transesophageal echocardiogram, the lack of opening of the aortic valve is due to:

    A. Aortic valve stenosis

    B. Low cardiac output

    C. A thrombus occluding the valve

Answers

ANSWER 1: C. The prodrome with skin and mucosal lesions are consistent with a viral myocarditis. The most common viruses associated with myocarditis are Coxsackievirus, influenza virus, adenovirus, echovirus, cytomegalovirus, and HIV.

The depressed myocardial function may be due to direct cytotoxicity via receptor-mediated entry of the virus into cardiac myocytes as well as an adverse autoimmune response to the infectious agent.

Clinical Course

The patient had clinical deterioration and had a left ventricular assist device placed.

Due to thrombosis and limb ischemia, the patient was taken to the operating room for revision of the external cannula.

A transesophageal echocardiogram was performed (Videos 20-5 and 20-6).

ANSWER 2: C. The very low cardiac output and stroke volume causes the valve to open only minimally and very briefly. In addition, due to the very low cardiac output, there is spontaneous contrast ("stasis") in the aortic root. This was a preterminal event, and the patient expired a few hours later.

A biopsy demonstrated lymphocytic infiltrate and necrosis consistent with acute viral myocarditis.

Suggested Reading

Felker GM, Boehmer JP, Hruban RH, et al. Echocardiographic findings in fulminant and acute myocarditis. *J Am Coll Cardiol.* 2000;36:227–232.

CASE 21

Acute Shortness of Breath following Surgery due to a Motor Vehicle Accident

A 40-year-old man had orthopedic surgery following a motor vehicle accident. He subsequently developed acute shortness of breath. Transthoracic echocardiogram images were obtained (Figs. 21-1 to 21-3 and Video 21-1).

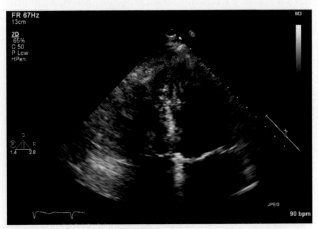

Figure 21-1.

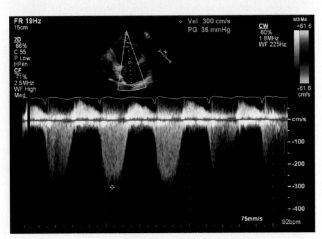

Figure 21-2.

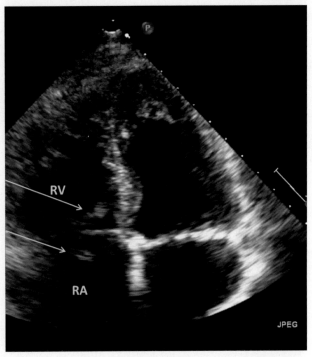

Figure 21-3.

QUESTION 1. The most likely diagnosis is:

A. Right ventricular (RV) stress cardiomyopathy

B. RV infarction

C. Fat embolus

D. Pulmonary embolism (PE) with clot from legs

QUESTION 2. RV echocardiographic predictors of outcome in acute pulmonary embolism include:

A. RV/left ventricular (LV) end-diastolic diameter ratio

B. Stress and strain rates

C. RV fractional area change

D. RV/LV end-diastolic diameter ratio and RV fractional area change

E. Stress and strain rates and RV fractional area change

QUESTION 3. True or False? RV dilatation occurs after an increase in pulmonary vascular resistance (PVR) in acute PE.

QUESTION 4. True or False? Regional RV wall motion abnormalities in PE are completely reversible.

Answers

ANSWER 1: D. The mass is shaped like a cast from the iliofemoral veins and is consistent with a clot "in transit" causing pulmonary emboli.

During the echocardiographic exam, the clot disappeared and embolized to the lungs (Video 21-2).

ANSWER 2: E. The RV/LV end-diastolic diameter ratio was shown to be a predictor of adverse clinical events and/or hospital survival in patients with acute pulmonary embolism.

RV fractional area change was found to be an independent predictor of heart failure, sudden death, stroke, and/or mortality in studies of patients after pulmonary embolism and myocardial infarction.

Stress and strain rates are less useful due to lack of normative data.

ANSWER 3: FALSE. Conditions that acutely increase PVR, such as pulmonary embolism, result in increases in RV size prior to the augmentation of pulmonary pressures, which ultimately may result in RV hypertrophy.

ANSWER 4: TRUE. Initial increases in RV volume and diameters are often accompanied by a specific pattern of abnormal regional wall motion in which the mid-RV free wall becomes hypo or dyskinetic with relative sparing or even a hyperkinetic RV apex as seen in Video 21-2. Regional RV wall motion abnormalities in PE are completely reversible with improvement in pulmonary hemodynamics.

Suggested Readings

Farfel Z, Shechter M, Vered Z, et al. Review of echocardiographically diagnosed right heart entrapment of pulmonary emboli-in-transit with emphasis on management. *Am Heart J.* 1987;113:171–178.

Rudski LG, Lai WW, Afilalo J, et al. Guidelines for the echocardiographic assessment of the right heart in adults: a report from the American Society of Echocardiography endorsed by the European Association of Echocardiography, a registered branch of the European Society of Cardiology, and the Canadian Society of Echocardiography. *J Am Soc Echocardiogr.* 2010;23(7):685–713.

CASE 22

Syncopal Event with a Bruised Sternum

A 41-year-old African American man presents after a syncopal event that occurred while driving a car. The patient was involved in a head-on collision and had a bruised sternum.

The physical exam is remarkable for a well-developed 41-year-old man in no acute distress. Neck veins are not elevated and carotid pulses are symmetric and normal in caliber. Lungs are clear to auscultation bilaterally. Cardiac exam reveals a point of maximum impulse displaced to the anterior axillary line. There is a normal S1 and S2 with no murmurs, rubs, or gallops. There is no peripheral edema.

An echocardiogram is ordered to assess left ventricular (LV) systolic function (Videos 22-1 to 22-4).

QUESTION 1. Which of the following studies should be performed to clarify the diagnosis?

- A. Repeat echocardiogram with LV contrast
- B. Myocardial perfusion single-photon emission computed tomography
- C. Coronary angiography
- D. Coronary computed tomographic angiography
- E. Tilt table test

QUESTION 2. After looking at Videos 22-5 to 22-7, what is the most likely etiology of cardiomyopathy?

- A. Ischemic heart disease
- B. Acute myocarditis
- C. Arrhythmogenic right ventricular (RV) dysplasia
- D. Noncompaction cardiomyopathy
- E. Hypertrophic cardiomyopathy

Answers

ANSWER 1: A. The patient has a markedly depressed LV systolic function with marked LV hypertrophy. Although working up ischemia with a myocardial perfusion study, coronary angiography, or coronary computed tomographic angiography may be indicated, the best first step would be to perform an echocardiogram with LV contrast (Videos 22-5 to 22-7). There is no indication for tilt table testing.

ANSWER 2: D. Noncompaction cardiomyopathy, also called spongiform cardiomyopathy, is a rare cardiomyopathy that results from the failure of myocardial development during embryogenesis. Noncompaction can be diagnosed on the basis of a ratio of noncompacted myocardium to compacted myocardium of 2:1 or greater. Microbubble contrast helps to separately visualize noncompacted myocardium, which allows contrast to freely travel within its sinusoids, from compacted myocardium, which has a more contrast-free appearance.

Suggested Reading

Captur G, Nihoyannopoulos P. Left ventricular non-compaction: genetic heterogeneity, diagnosis and clinical course. *Int J Cardiol.* 2010;140:145–153.

Weight Loss and Low-Grade Fevers

A 41-year-old man was admitted to the hospital with a 1-month history of fatigue, shortness of breath, weight loss, and low-grade fevers.

On physical examination, he is ill-appearing. He has a blood pressure of 119/56 mm Hg, heart rate of 123 beats per minute, respiratory rate of 18 breaths per minute, temperature of 100.8°F; and his oxygen saturation is 97%. He has bounding (3+) peripheral pulses, a 1/6 systolic ejection murmur, and 1/4 diastolic murmur at the apex as well as a gallop.

Computed tomography (CT) scan revealed a splenic infarction versus a mass. Blood cultures were also obtained.

See Videos 23-1 to 23-3.

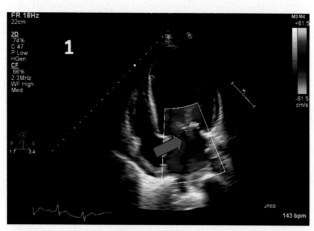

Figure 23-1.

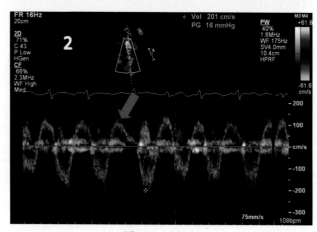

Figure 23-2.

QUESTION 1. Which of the following are true?

A. There is a bicuspid aortic valve with mild aortic regurgitation (AR)

B. There is a trileaflet aortic valve with severe AR

C. There is a bicuspid aortic valve with severe AR

D. There is an aortic valve vegetation

E. There is a bicuspid aortic valve with severe AR and an aortic valve vegetation

QUESTION 2. Additional transthoracic images are performed. Shown are color Doppler (Fig. 23-1) and pulse Doppler (Fig. 23-2) images. What is the significance of the Doppler findings in the figures?

A. There is severe mitral regurgitation (MR)

B. There is mild MR

C. There is severe AR

D. None of the options

QUESTION 3. The patient develops hypoxic hypercapnic respiratory failure requiring intubation. A transesophageal echocardiogram (TEE) is performed (Videos 23-4 to 23-8).

Based on the TEE findings:

A. You initiate antibiotic therapy

B. You call for surgical consultation the next day

C. You arrange for emergent aortic valve replacement

D. You send the patient for a CT scan to rule out aortic dissection

E. You initiate antibiotic therapy and arrange for emergent aortic valve replacement

Answers

ANSWER 1: E. The aortic valve is bicuspid with a raphe between the right and left coronary cusp, at times creating the illusion of a trileaflet aortic valve. The aortic valve is thickened with evidence of vegetation and damage of the cusps in the long-axis view. The color Doppler shows wide open AR with diastolic MR.

ANSWER 2: C. There is evidence of severe AR. Figure 23-3, using color Doppler, demonstrates the presence of diastolic MR, which is seen with severe acute AR and is associated with severely elevated left ventricular end-diastolic pressure. Figure 23-4 depicts the pulse wave Doppler finding of holodiastolic flow reversal in the descending aorta consistent with severe AR.

ANSWER 3: E. The findings are consistent with acute severe AR and emergent surgical repair is indicated because of rapid clinical deterioration.

In addition, there is tachycardia and preclosure of the mitral valve as well as diastolic MR all indicative of acute severe AR. Blood cultures from a minimum of two sites should be obtained and antibiotics should be started.

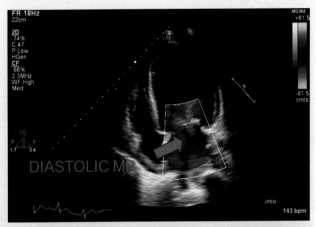

Figure 23-3.

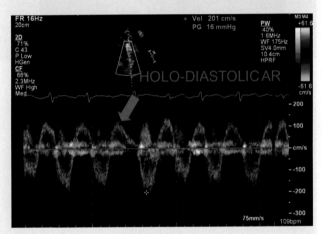

Figure 23-4.

Answers

SUBSEQUENT FINDINGS

Surgical findings show aortic valve endocarditis (Figs. 23-5 to 23-7).

Cultures from the blood and valve tissue grew *Streptococcus Abiotrophia*.

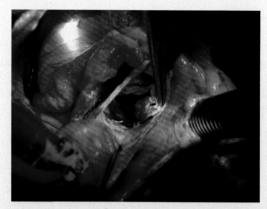

Figure 23-6.

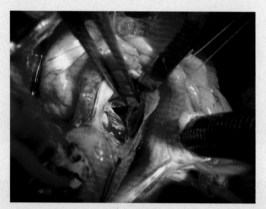

Figure 23-5.

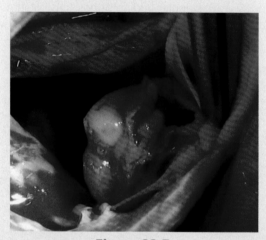

Figure 23-7.

Suggested Reading

Vogt PR, von Segesser LK, Jenni R, et al. Emergency surgery for acute infective aortic valve endocarditis: performance of cryopreserved homografts and mode of failure. *Eur J Cardiothorac Surg.* 1997;11:53–61.

Atrial Fibrillation and Shortness of Breath

A 42-year-old woman had her first episode of atrial fibrillation 3 years ago. Over the last year, she developed symptoms of fatigue and shortness of breath.

Physical examination showed no signs of cardiac decompensation. On auscultation, a split second heart sound was noted.

See Figures 24-1 to 24-3 and Videos 24-1 and 24-2.

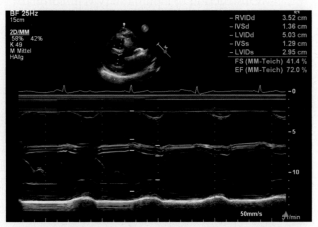

Figure 24-1. M-mode, parasternal long-axis view.

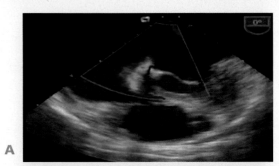

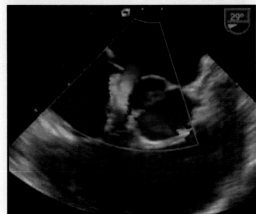

Figure 24-2. A. Conventional 2D transesophageal echocardiogram (TEE) with color Doppler in different planes at 0°. **B.** Conventional 2D TEE with color Doppler at 30°.

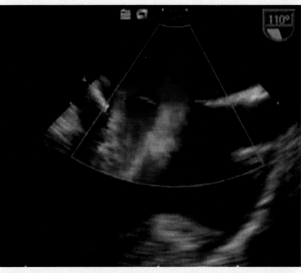

Figure 24-3. Conventional 2D TEE with and without color Doppler at 110°.

QUESTION 1. What is the diagnosis?

    A. Ventricular septal defect

    B. Secundum atrial septal defect

    C. Atrioventricular (AV) canal defect

    D. Left-to-right shunting through a stretched patent foramen ovale

QUESTION 2. How would you proceed?

A. The patient has only mild symptoms; a routine follow-up in 6 months is sufficient
B. Closure of the atrial septal defects (surgery or transcatheter closure)

QUESTION 3. What has to be judged after device positioning?

A. Device position
    - Device position has to be stable
    - Both disks should be opposed to the septum secundum
B. Residual shunt/additional defects
C. Complications
    - Pericardial effusion
    - Obstruction of a pulmonary vein/coronary sinus
    - Disturbance of AV–valve function
    - Thrombi
D. All of the options

Answers

ANSWER 1: B. The short-axis view (Fig. 24-2 and Video 24-1) at 30° shows that the patient had no aortic rim, and the long-axis view (Fig. 24-3 and Video 24-2) at 110° documents two atrial septal defects in the secundum portion of the atrial septum.

ANSWER 2: B. Indications for atrial septal defect closure include symptoms and/or right ventricular/right atrial enlargement and/or a pulmonic blood flow: Systemic blood flow > 1.5 and/or paradoxical embolism.[1]

The patient has symptoms, and the M-mode (Fig. 24-1) shows right ventricular enlargement.

Therefore, treatment is indicated, and it was decided to close the defect with percutaneous closure devices.

The procedural steps are shown in Figures 24-4 to 24-6 and Video 24-3.

Right heart catheterization documented a relevant shunt, and the additive measurements of both defects were larger than 40 mm. Therefore, the defects could not be closed with a single device, and two devices had to be implanted.

The procedural steps are shown in Figures 24-5 and 24-6 and Video 24-3.

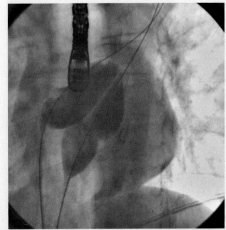

- Right heart catheterization: Qp: Qs 1.9
- Ballon sizing caudal defect: 18 mm
- Ballon sizing cranial defect: 23 mm

2 Amplatzer extra stiff wires and
2 sizing balloons (40 mm – Numed/NMT) are placed in the defects

Figure 24-4. Right heart catheterization and measurements with balloon sizing.

Answers

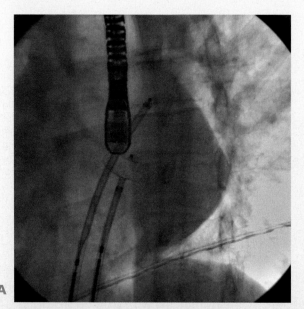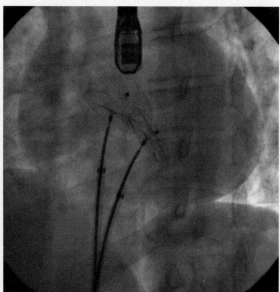

Figure 24-5. **A.** Two Amplatzer delivery sheath can be seen: one is positioned in the caudal (9 F) and the other in the cranial defect (10 F). **B.** The placement of a 18-mm and a 24-mm Amplatzer septal occluder is shown.

ANSWER 3: **D.** Stable device position, closure of the defect with no residual shunt, and lack of procedural complications are all part of the postprocedural assessment. See Video 24-4 to 24-6 and Figures 24-7 to 24-9, which demonstrate what needs to be assessed after device positioning.

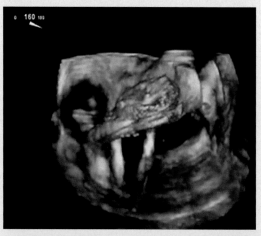

Figure 24-6. Assessment before device release. 3D TEE zoom: Both occluders are positioned but still attached to the delivery cables. The caudal occluder is "sandwiched" in between the disks of the larger cranial defect.

Answers

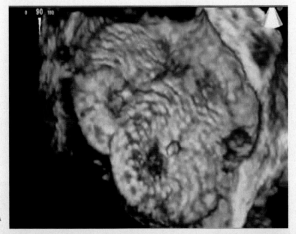
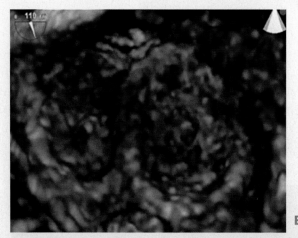

Figure 24-7. Six-month follow up. The 3D TEE zoom images show a left atrial (**A**) and a right atrial (**B**) view of the occluders.

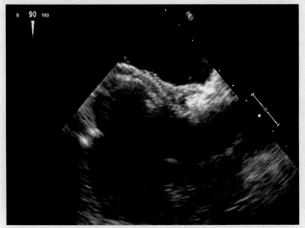
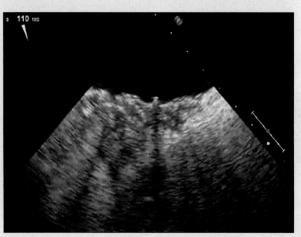

Figure 24-8. Six-month follow up. 2D TEE 90° view: The position of both occluders is shown. At the 6-month follow up, she no longer had dyspnea and experienced an improvement in functional capacity.

Figure 24-9. In this image, complete closure is confirmed by administration of agitated saline intravenously during a Valsalva maneuver.

Reference

1. Warnes CA, Williams RG, Bashore TM, et al. Atrial septal defect. In: ACC/AHA 2008 guidelines for the management of adults with congenital heart disease. *J Am Coll Cardiol.* 2008;52(23):e173–e178.

CASE 25

Marfan Syndrome with Sharp Chest Pain

*T*he patient is a 43-year-old woman with a history of Marfan syndrome. She had a Bentall procedure 10 years ago with a composite Dacron graft (INVISTA, North Wichita, Kansas) replacing the native ascending aorta and a mechanical St. Jude Medical aortic valve (St. Jude Medical, St. Paul, Minnesota). The patient now presents complaining of sharp chest pains worse not only with inspiration but also with firm palpation. An echocardiogram was done to further evaluate the patient's chest pain (Videos 25-1 to 25-3 and Figs. 25-1 to 25-3).

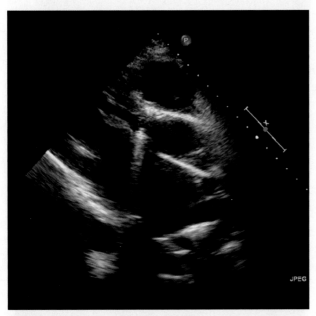

Figure 25-1.

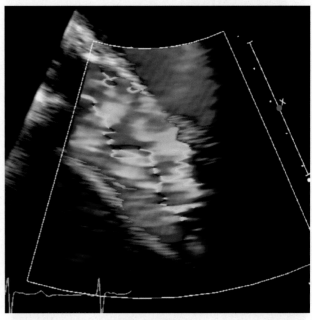

Figure 25-3.

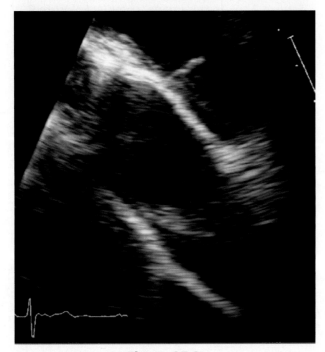

Figure 25-2.

QUESTION 1. The transthoracic echocardiogram demonstrates:

    A. An ascending aortic dissection

    B. An artifact

    C. A malfunctioning aortic valve

    D. None of the options

QUESTION 2. Which do you recommend?

    A. Emergent aortic surgery

    B. An invasive aortogram and coronary angiogram

    C. No further evaluation

    D. A computed tomography (CT) angiogram or magnetic resonance imaging (MRI)

Answers

ANSWER 1: D. The echocardiogram shows a mobile linear echo density within the Dacron aortic root graft. No definitive diagnosis can be made based on these images.

ANSWER 2: D. Further evaluation with a CT or MRI is warranted to get a better assessment of the endolumen of the graft and a 3D reconstruction to facilitate the diagnosis.

   The echo abnormality is due to a kink (Fig. 25-4, *arrow*) in the aortic graft which moves in and out of plane with each cardiac cycle, giving the appearance of a dissection flap, which would be unlikely in a Dacron graft.

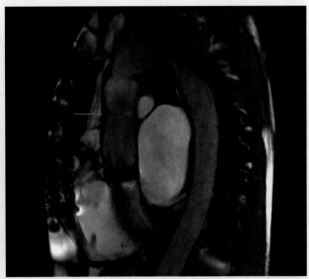

Figure 25-4.

Reference

1. Al-Mohaissen M, Skarsgard P, Khoo C, et al. Expanding arch aneurysm causing a "kink" in a Bentall graft and heart failure. *J Thorac Imaging*. 2012;27:W88–W90.

CASE 26

Worsening Dyspnea on Exertion and Reduced Exercise Capacity

A 44-year-old woman presents with a 6-month history of worsening dyspnea on exertion. She has reduced exercise capacity and has to stop to rest after walking one to two blocks.

On physical exam, her blood pressure is 125/76 mm Hg, and her pulse is 72 beats per minute and regular. Neck veins are flat. Carotid pulses are bounding. Lungs are clear to auscultation bilaterally. Cardiac exam reveals a hyperdynamic apical impulse in the fifth intercostal space, midclavicular line. There is a 3/6 systolic nonradiating ejection murmur in the left upper sternal border. Extremities are warm with no peripheral edema.

Echocardiography is performed to evaluate left ventricular systolic function (Video 26-1).

QUESTION 1. On the parasternal long-axis view, there is evidence of enlargement of what?

A. Aortic root
B. Right ventricle
C. Coronary sinus
D. Left atrium
E. Coronary sinus and left atrium

QUESTION 2. See Videos 26-2 to 26-4. The large tubular structures surrounding the heart are most likely:

A. Hydatid cysts
B. Cysticerci
C. Coronary arteries
D. Engorged pulmonary veins
E. None of the choices

Answers

ANSWER 1: E. Both the coronary sinus and the left atrium are enlarged. The coronary sinus lies within the left atrioventricular groove and is visualized just posterior to the mitral annulus within the pericardial space. It is usually less than 1 cm in diameter, but in this patient, it is nearly 3 cm in diameter.

ANSWER 2: C. The engorged structures are the patient's own coronary arteries. This patient has a coronary arteriovenous fistula with left-to-right shunting and high-output congestive heart failure. The high-flow state that occurs with this condition causes enlargement of all the coronary arteries and cardiac veins.

Suggested Reading

Luo L, Kebede S, Wu S, et al. Coronary artery fistulae. *Am J Med Sci.* 2006;332:79–84.

CASE 27

Transient Ischemic Attack

A 44-year-old woman suffered from a transient ischemic attack 2 years ago. An echocardiogram revealed a patent foramen ovale (PFO) in association with an atrial septal aneurysm. No other cause for her ischemic cerebral event could be determined. Therefore, she underwent PFO closure, and a 20-mm Premere device (Velocimed LLC, Minneapolis, Minnesota) was implanted uneventfully. Aspirin (100 mg) daily and clopidogrel (75 mg) daily were prescribed after the procedure.

At her first follow-up echocardiogram, the device position appeared appropriate, and there was no residual shunt through the PFO. However, a small thrombus was seen attached to the right atrial side of the Premere occluder. This is shown in the following image in a long-axis view (live 3D transesophageal echocardiogram [TEE]). (See Fig. 27-1 and Video 27-1.)

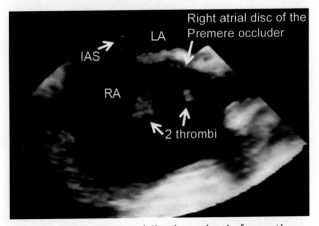

Figure 27-1. Two mobile thrombotic formations attached to the right atrial side of the Premere occluder (*IAS*, interatrial septum; *LA*, left atrium; *RA*, right atrium).

QUESTION 1. Which therapy would you recommend to treat the thrombus?

  A. Continue with aspirin and clopidogrel and perform another follow-up TEE in 4 to 6 weeks
  B. Anticoagulation therapy
  C. Anticoagulation therapy and aspirin
  D. Anticoagulation therapy, aspirin, and clopidogrel
  E. Surgery

QUESTION 2. A follow-up echocardiogram showed that the thrombus enlarged to a size of 20 x 20 mm even under full anticoagulation therapy in combination with aspirin. Which further strategy would you suggest according to your echocardiogram findings?

  A. Continue with anticoagulation therapy and aspirin and perform another TEE in 6 weeks
  B. Add clopidogrel to anticoagulation therapy and aspirin
  C. Send the patient to surgery

Answers

ANSWER 1: C. The overall incidence of thrombus occurrence after transcatheter PFO closure is rare.

Currently, there are no accepted guidelines regarding the best management strategy in case of a thrombus on a device.

In our case, full anticoagulation therapy in combination with aspirin was administered.

The following 3D TEE full volume image shows the situation 2 months later (Fig. 27-2 and Video 27-2).

The thrombus enlarged to a size of 20 × 20 mm even under full anticoagulation therapy in combination with aspirin.

No embolic events occurred.

Coagulation disorders were excluded, and thus this represents a case where aspirin was found not to be effective in preventing thrombus formation in this patient.

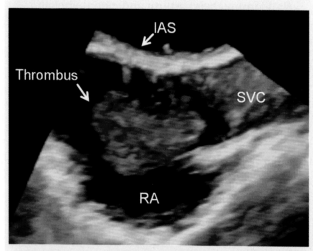

Figure 27-2. Thrombotic mass attached to the right atrial side of the Premere occluder (*IAS*, interatrial septum; *RA*, right atrium; *SVC*, superior vena cava).

ANSWER 2: C. Again, there is no accepted "best practice" or guidelines available to guide treatment.

According to the large size of the thrombus (Fig. 27-3), the decision was made to remove the thrombotic mass.

Intraoperatively, it was shown that the thrombus was attached to a part of the release string of the Premere occluder.

Therefore, this part was removed, and the occluder was left in place (Fig. 27-4 and Video 27-3).

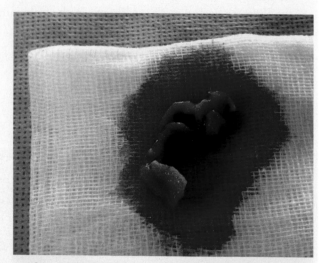

Figure 27-3. The removed thrombotic mass is shown in this image.

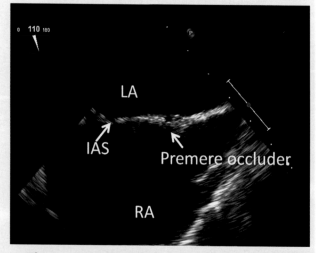

Figure 27-4. 2D TEE 6 weeks after thrombus removal. No recurrence of thrombus formation could be detected.

Reference

1. Krumsdorf U, Ostermayer S, Billinger K, et al. Incidence and clinical course of thrombus formation on atrial septal defect and patent foramen ovale closure devices in 1.000 consecutive patients. *J Am Col Cardiol.* 2004;43:302–309.

CASE 28

Atrial Fibrillation, Dyspnea with Heavy Exertion

*T*he patient is a 47-year-old man with a history of atrial fibrillation. Eleven months prior to the transthoracic echocardiogram, he underwent a prolonged atrial fibrillation ablation procedure. He now returns complaining of dyspnea with heavy exertion. A transesophageal echocardiogram is done to further evaluate his dyspnea (Fig. 28-1).

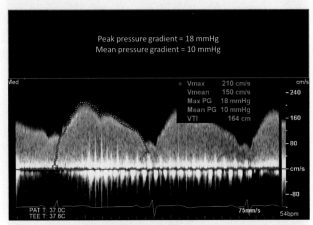

Figure 28-1.

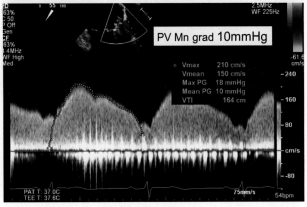

Figure 28-2.

QUESTION 1. What does the Doppler show?

- A. The mitral inflow suggests mitral stenosis (MS)
- B. There is MS and mitral regurgitation
- C. This is a normal pulmonary vein flow
- D. This is consistent with pulmonary vein stenosis

QUESTION 2. True or False? The aliased color velocities come from the pulmonary vein (Fig. 28-2).

QUESTION 3. Why might there be pulmonary vein stenosis?

- A. Congenital
- B. Atrial fibrillation ablation

Answers

ANSWER 1: D. The Doppler shows pulmonary vein stenosis (Fig. 28-3 and Video 28-1).

ANSWER 2: TRUE.

ANSWER 3: B. Atrial fibrillation ablation can lead to pulmonary vein stenosis due to thermal or cryoablation damage, which can shrink the pulmonary vein.

In addition, this patient (Fig. 28-4) had a Watchman closure device (*arrow*) for occlusion of the left atrial appendage. This device could potentially obstruct the left pulmonary vein. However, the gradient occurred after atrial fibrillation ablation and before the Watchman device was inserted.

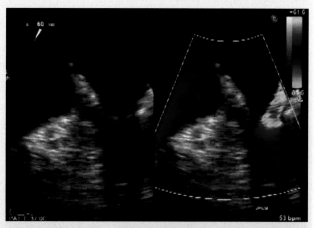

Figure 28-3.

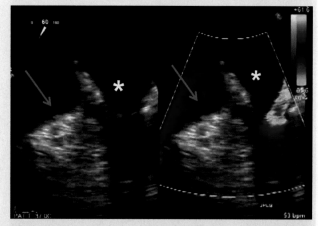

Figure 28-4. Left upper pulmonary vein (*asterisk*).

Suggested Reading

Stavrakis S, Madden GW, Stoner JA, et al. Transesophageal echocardiography for the diagnosis of pulmonary vein stenosis after catheter ablation of atrial fibrillation: a systematic review. *Echocardiography*. 2010;27:1141–1146.

CASE 29

Preparation for Kidney Donation

A 48-year-old healthy man is referred for a stress echocardiogram in preparation for kidney donation. A mass is noted in the right atrium moving between the right atrium and the right ventricle during the cardiac cycle (Fig. 29-1 and Video 29-1.)

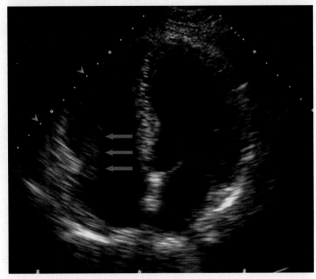

Figure 29-1.

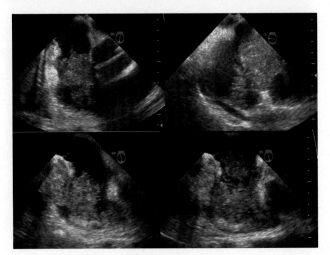

Figure 29-2.

QUESTION 1. What should you do next?

A. Start anticoagulation; the mass is probably a thrombus

B. Perform a transesophageal echocardiogram (TEE) to further evaluate the mass

C. Send off blood cultures to work the patient up for endocarditis

D. Nothing for now. The mass is probably benign and is on the right side so no risk of stroke

QUESTION 2. See Figure 29-2 and Videos 29-2 to 29-5. What is a likely diagnosis after these TEE images?

A. Endocarditis

B. Right atrial (RA) myxoma

C. Thrombus in transit

D. RA sarcoma

E. Metastatic disease to the right atrium

Answers

ANSWER 1: B. Although blood cultures could be considered, there is no history of constitutional symptoms or intravenous drug abuse, and endocarditis is unlikely. In situ thrombus would be unlikely, given the patient does not have atrial fibrillation. A mass should never be ignored, and a TEE will better delineate the structure as to size and attachment and so forth. A valvular lesion would raise suspicion for endocarditis, and a thrombus in transit from a venous leg or pelvic structure could be better identified with the TEE. Additional lesions in other areas of the heart may also be detected and aid in diagnosis. Furthermore, a lesion of this size should be considered for surgical removal, and the surgeons would need to have more information from the TEE before planning the surgery.

ANSWER 2: D. Figure 29-3 and Videos 29-3 and 29-4 demonstrates a large heterogeneous mass in the right atrium (*single asterisk*) that has invaded through the atrial wall (*arrows*), and the mass is seen to involve the pericardial and extra cardiac space (*double asterisk*). The location of the mass and the fact that it has invaded the tissues increases the likelihood that this is a malignant lesion, most likely sarcoma. The mass was excised, and pathology confirming angiosarcoma is shown in Figure 29-4.

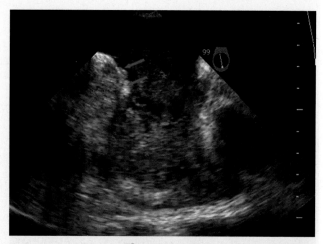

Figure 29-3.

Answers

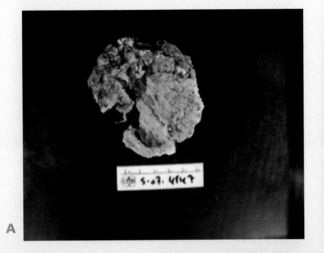

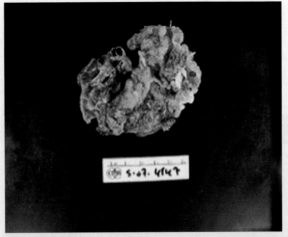

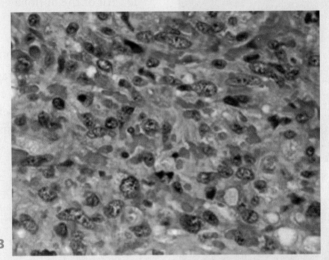

Figure 29-4A,B. High-grade angiosarcoma.

Suggested Readings

Butany J, Nair V, Naseemuddin A, et al. Cardiac tumors: diagnosis and management. *Lancet Oncol.* 2005;6(4):219–228.

Orlandi A, Ferlosio A, Roselli M, et al. Cardiac sarcomas: an update. *J Thorac Oncol.* 2010;5(9):1483–1489.

Yang HS, Sengupta S, Umland MM, et al. Primary cardiac angiosarcoma evaluated with contrast two-dimensional and real-time three-dimensional echocardiography. *Eur J Echocardiogr.* 2008;9:733–738.

Jugular Venous Distension, Tachycardia, and Borderline Hypotension

A 48-year-old man complains of shortness of breath and fatigue. He has jugular venous distension, tachycardia (heart rate of 108 to 124 beats per minute), and borderline hypotension with a systolic blood pressure of 90 mm Hg. See Videos 30-1 and 30-2 and Figures 30-1 and 30-2.

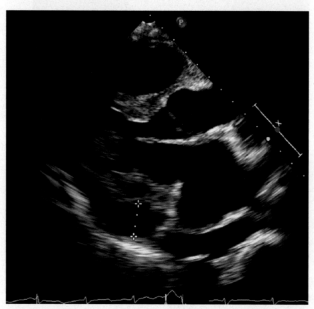

Figure 30-1.

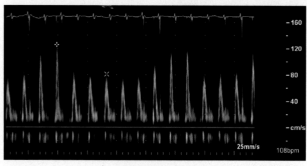

Figure 30-2.

QUESTION 1. The echocardiogram Doppler studies demonstrate:

   A. Posterior pericardial effusion
   B. Doppler mitral inflow tracing consistent with pericardial tamponade
   C. Large, bilateral pleural effusions
   D. All of the options

QUESTION 2. You recommend:

   A. Computed tomography or magnetic resonance imaging to further evaluate for tamponade
   B. Urgent pericardiocentesis
   C. Urgent thoracentesis

Answers

ANSWER 1: D. A respiratory variation of > 25% in Doppler mitral inflow is consistent with pericardial tamponade. There is a posterior pericardial effusion and large, bilateral pleural effusions.

ANSWER 2: C. Large pleural effusions can result in hemodynamics and a Doppler mitral inflow pattern exactly like tamponade due to pericardial fluid accumulation. A thoracentesis should be done first (Video 30-3 and Fig. 30-3); if there is still evidence of tamponade physiology on echo, a pericardiocentesis can be reconsidered.

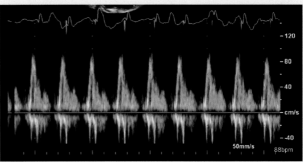

Figure 30-3. Postthoracentesis, the patient's systolic blood pressure rose to 110 mm Hg, pulse rate dropped to 88 beats per minute, and, as shown here, the Doppler mitral inflow tracing normalized with resolution of the respiratory variation. Thus, the patient's finding of "pericardial tamponade" resolved with thoracentesis.

Suggested Reading

Kaplan LM, Epstein SK, Schwartz SL, et al. Clinical, echocardiographic, and hemodynamic evidence of cardiac tamponade caused by large pleural effusions. *Am J Respir Crit Care Med.* 1995;151:904–908.

Antiphospholipid Antibody Syndrome

A 50-year-old woman with a history of antiphospholipid antibody syndrome, a history of ST segment elevation (Q wave) myocardial infarction involving the left anterior descending artery, history of recurrent deep vein thrombosis status post inferior vena cava filter, and who is status post mitral valve replacement presents with 1 week of increasing dyspnea on exertion, now with dyspnea at rest. Her prescribed medications include fondaparinux and clopidogrel. A transthoracic echocardiogram is performed (Figs. 31-1 to 31-3), followed by a 3D transesophageal echocardiogram (Figs. 31-4 and 31-5).

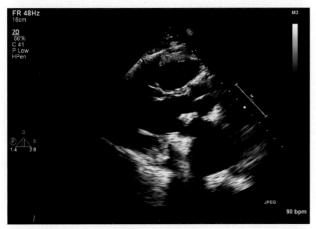

Figure 31-1.

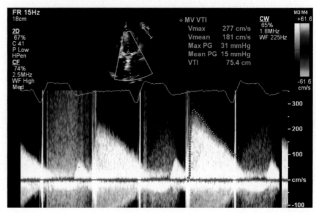

Figure 31-3.

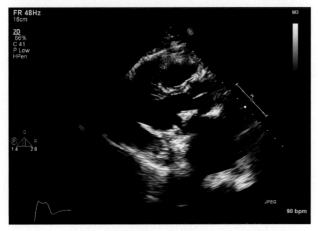

Figure 31-2.

QUESTION 1. The recommended treatment for this condition is:

    A. Immediate surgery

    B. Fibrinolytics

    C. Plasmapheresis

    D. Pulse steroids

    E. More than one of the choices

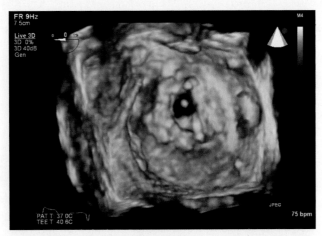

Figure 31-4.

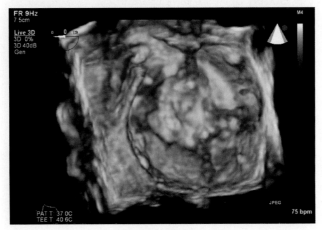

Figure 31-5.

QUESTION 2. This patient has the following type of valve:

    A. Bioprosthetic mitral valve

    B. Starr-Edwards caged-ball valve

    C. Bileaflet mechanical valve

    D. None of the options

QUESTION 3. The following is the *most likely* normal range of transmitral gradients for this type of valve:

    A. Peak, 10 to 12; mean, 2.5 to 5 mm Hg

    B. Peak, 17 to 20; mean, 8 to 12 mm Hg

    C. Peak, 5 to 10; mean, 1 to 2 mm Hg

    D. None of the options

Answers

ANSWER 1: E. This patient has thrombosis of her prosthetic mitral valve. There is no consensus among the major societies for initial therapy for prosthetic valve thrombosis (PVT). Furthermore, in this case—and not addressed in the guidelines—is the value of steroids and plasmapheresis in the treatment of PVT associated with antiphospholipid antibody syndrome.[1]

The various guideline recommendations for PVT are summarized here:

- American College of Cardiology/American Heart Association[2]:
  Fibrinolytic therapy for a left-sided prosthetic valve obstructed by thrombus is associated with significant risks (cerebral emboli in 12% to 15% of cases) and is often ineffective. Fibrinolytic therapy in such patients is reserved for those in whom surgical intervention carries a high risk and those with contraindications to surgery. In patients with a "small clot" who are in NYHA functional class I or II, treatment with short-term intravenous UFH therapy or continuous infusion of fibrinolytic therapy may be considered.
- European Society of Cardiology[3]:
  Surgery as first-line treatment regardless of clinical status and thrombus size however, fibrinolysis should be considered in:
  - Critically ill patients unlikely to survive surgery because of comorbidities or severely impaired cardiac function before developing valve thrombosis.
  - Situations in which surgery is not immediately available and the patient cannot be transferred.
  - Thrombosis of tricuspid or pulmonary valve replacements, because of the higher success rate and low risk of systemic embolism.
- American College of Chest Physicians[4]:
  Thrombolysis for all right-sided valves and for left-sided valves iv thrombus is < 0.8 cm². For patients with left-sided PVT and large thrombus area (> 0.8 cm²), emergency surgery should be considered. If surgery is not available or considered high risk, they suggest fibrinolytic therapy.
- Society of Heart Valve Disease[5]:
  Thrombolysis is the first-line treatment for obstructive PVT, independent of NYHA class and thrombus size if there are no contraindications.

ANSWER 2: C. The patient has a bileaflet St. Jude mitral valve and one of the leaflets is not moving due to a thrombosis.

ANSWER 3: A. Depending on the ring size, normal mechanical bileaflet mitral valve gradients average peak, 7 to 15; mean, 2 to 6 mm Hg.

References

1. Espinosa G, Bucciarelli S, Cervera R, et al. Thrombotic microangiopathic haemolytic anaemia and antiphospholipid antibodies. *Ann Rheum Dis.* 2004;63:730–736.
2. Bonow RO, Carabello BA, Chatterjee K, et al. 2008 focused update incorporated into the ACC/AHA 2006 guidelines for the management of patients with valvular heart disease: a report of the American College of Cardiology/American Heart Association Task Force on Practice Guidelines (Writing Committee to revise the 1998 guidelines for the management of patients with valvular heart disease). Endorsed by the Society of Cardiovascular Anesthesiologists, Society for Cardiovascular Angiography and Interventions, and Society of Thoracic Surgeons. *J Am Coll Cardiol.* 2008;52:e1–e142.
3. Joint Task Force on the Management of Valvular Heart Disease of the European Society of Cardiology (ESC), European Association for Cardio-Thoracic Surgery (EACTS), Vahanian A, et al. Guidelines on the management of valvular heart disease (version 2012). *Eur Heart J.* 2012;33:2451–2496.
4. Salem DN, O'Gara PT, Madias C, et al. American College of Chest Physicians. Valvular and structural heart disease: American College of Chest Physicians evidence-based clinical practice guidelines (8th edition). *Chest.* 2008;133:593S–629S.
5. Lengyel M, Horstkotte D, Völler H, et al. Working Group Infection, Thrombosis, Embolism and Bleeding of the Society for Heart Valve Disease. Recommendations for the management of prosthetic valve thrombosis. *J Heart Valve Dis.* 2005;14:567–575.

Suggested Reading

Zoghbi WA, Chambers JB, Dumesnil JG, et al. Recommendations for evaluation of prosthetic valves with echocardiography and Doppler ultrasound: a report from the American Society of Echocardiography's Guidelines and Standards Committee and the Task Force on Prosthetic Valves, developed in conjunction with the American College of Cardiology Cardiovascular Imaging Committee, Cardiac Imaging Committee of the American Heart Association, the European Association of Echocardiography, a registered branch of the European Society of Cardiology, the Japanese Society of Echocardiography and the Canadian Society of Echocardiography, endorsed by the American College of Cardiology Foundation, American Heart Association, European Association of Echocardiography, a registered branch of the European Society of Cardiology, the Japanese Society of Echocardiography, and Canadian Society of Echocardiography. *J Am Soc Echocardiogr.* 2009;22:975–1014.

CASE 32

Closure of Patent Foramen Ovale

A 52-year-old woman had a closure of a patent foramen ovale (PFO) with a 30-mm Helex septal occluder (W. L. Gore & Associates, Flagstaff, Arizona) after a left hemispheric stroke and recurrent transient ischemic attacks (TIAs).

She reported no further TIAs after the implantation.

At a 6-month follow-up transesophageal echocardiogram (TEE) after PFO closure, Figures 32-1 to 32-3 and Videos 32-1 to 32-3 were obtained to confirm device position.

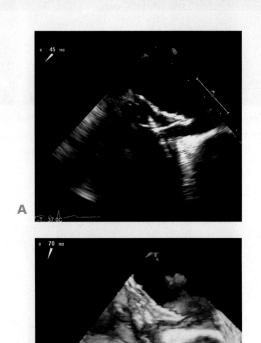

Figure 32-1. **A.** 2D TEE 45°. **B.** 3D TEE full-volume acquisition.

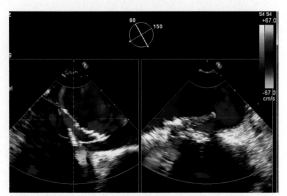

Figure 32-2. 2D TEE: X-plane (60° and 150°) with color Doppler.

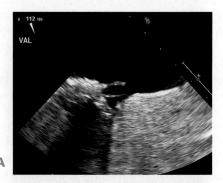

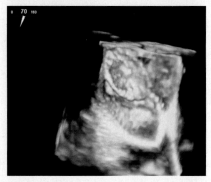

Figure 32-3. **A.** 2D TEE: Long-axis (LAX) view (112°) contrast study: Administration of agitated saline via a cubital vein. **B.** 3D TEE enface view from the left atrial (LA) side.

QUESTION 1. Based on Figures 32-1 to 32-3 and Videos 32-1 to 32-3, what is your diagnosis?

- A. The septum secundum is sealed adequately by the left and right atrial discs of the Helex septal occluder
- B. No complications after device implantation can be detected
- C. A complication after device closure can be verified
- D. A residual shunt can be detected

Answers

ANSWER 1: C. The images (Fig. 32-1 and Video 32-1) demonstrate that the septum secundum is not adequately sealed by the left and right atrial discs; a gap is seen along the septum secundum. The color flow (Fig. 32-2 and Video 32-2) clearly documents a residual shunt in this region, which has to be considered a complication.

In the contrast study (Fig. 32-3A and Video 32-3A), an atypical LA tissue bridge can be seen while the probe is turned. This tissue bridge prevents the LA disc from sealing the interatrial septum (IAS).

The 3D TEE enface view (Fig. 32-3B and Video 32-3B) confirms these findings: the LA disc is trapped and kept away from the IAS by this atypical tissue bridge as seen in Figure 32-4.

The Helex septal occluder is composed of a super elastic, spiral-shaped, single-strand nitinol wire covered with a biocompatible membrane composed of expanded polytetrafluoroethylene. After release from the sheath, the wire assumes a spiral shape. It consists of two circular, equally sized discs, fixed by an integral locking system passing through the center of the device from left to right. This locking system connects the atrial discs at their centers and stabilizes the occluder in the defect.

A multicenter experience in 128 patients with previous paradoxical embolism undergoing PFO closure with the Helex septal occluder reported complete closure in 90% of patients at a mean follow-up of 21 ± 11 months with no recurrent embolic events and no device-related thrombus formation.[1]

Across studies, a trend toward increased events related to residual leaks can be seen.[2]

Due to the mechanical problem causing the residual shunt in this case, it cannot be expected that the residual shunt will decrease over time.

Therefore, the patient underwent a second closure procedure with a 20-mm Premere device.

Figure 32-5 and Video 32-4 document complete closure after placement of a second device.

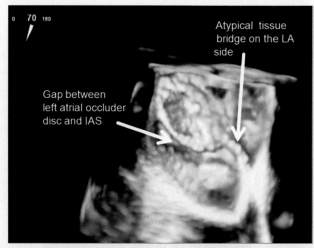

Figure 32-4. 3D enface view from the LA side: The occluder is separated from the septum by the atypical left LA bridge (*LA*, left atrium; *IAS*, interatrial septum).

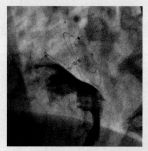

Figure 32-5. Flouroscopic image after placement of a second device (20-mm Premere occluder [Velocimed LLC, Minneapolis, Minnesota]). Contrast injection confirms complete closure.

References

1. Billinger K, Ostermeyer S, Carminati M, et al. HELEX Septal Occluder for transcatheter closure of patent foramen ovale: multicenter experience. *Euro Interv.* 2006;1:465–471.
2. Wahl A, Meier B, Haxel B, et al. Prognosis after percutaneous closure of patent foramen ovale for paradoxical embolism. *Neurology.* 2001;57:1330–1332.

Familial Hyperlipidemia and Exertional Chest Pain

A 52-year-old woman with familial hyperlipidemia complains of exertional chest pain but walks 2 to 5 miles daily without difficulty. She is feeling depressed and has had weight gain.

She has a 12-lead electrocardiogram (ECG) as depicted in Figure 33-1 and undergoes a supine bicycle stress echocardiogram with imaging at rest (heart rate [HR] 52 beats per minute; Videos 33-1 and 33-2), at intermediate exercise (HR 90 beats per minute; Videos 33-3 and 33-4), and during peak stress (HR 131 beats per minute = 78% maximum predicted HR; Videos 33-5 and 33-6), end-systolic frames depicted. Left ventricular ejection fraction is normal at rest without wall motion abnormalities (Fig. 33-2).

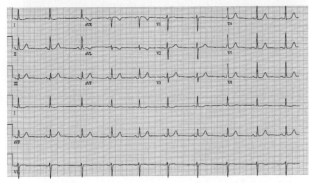

Figure 33-1. Resting 12-lead ECG.

QUESTION 1. Which statement is true?

A. The left ventricle (LV) is smallest at the intermediate stage exercise, suggesting a hibernating myocardium at rest

B. The LV cavity dilates at peak stress in a uniform pattern, suggesting a nonischemic cardiomyopathy

C. The LV cavity dilates in a regional pattern during peak stress, suggesting an ischemic response to stress

4-chamber views

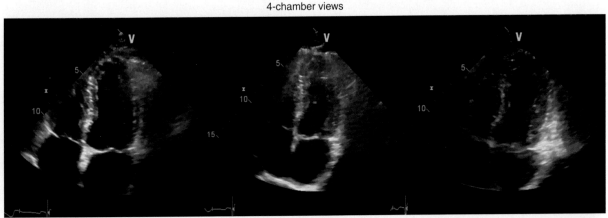

Baseline   Intermediate   Peak

2-chamber views

Figure 33-2A,B.

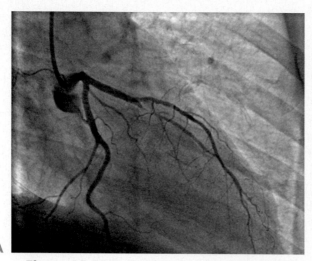
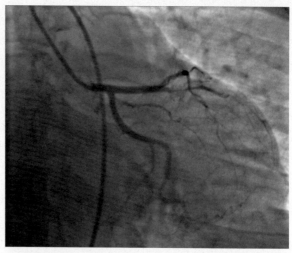

Figure 33-3A,B. Angiogram showing significant left anterior descending (LAD) disease after a large diagonal branch.

QUESTION 2. See Figure 33-3. The regional abnormality is consistent with:

A. Mid-LAD artery disease
B. Left main disease
C. Large, dominant right coronary artery disease
D. Left circumflex disease (LCx)
E. LAD and LCx

Answers

ANSWER 1: C. It is correct that the LV is smallest during intermediate stage exercise. This is a normal response to exercise, and in a patient with normal LV systolic function to start does not imply a hibernating myocardium. Our patient has regional variation in myocardial contractility during peak stress (Fig. 33-4), consistent with obstructive coronary artery disease. A patient with global LV dilatation at stress may have a nonischemic cardiomyopathy, significant valvular disease, or may have ischemic disease due to left main or triple vessel disease.

ANSWER 2: A. The images demonstrate distal lateral, apical and distal anterior, and inferior hypocontractility at peak stress (appearing as dilatation compared with intermediate stage exercise) consistent with a mid-LAD lesion. A dominant right coronary artery typically supplies the basal- to mid-inferior wall and inferior interventricular septum and portion of the posterior wall. The LCx supplies the basal- to mid-lateral wall and portion of the posterior wall.

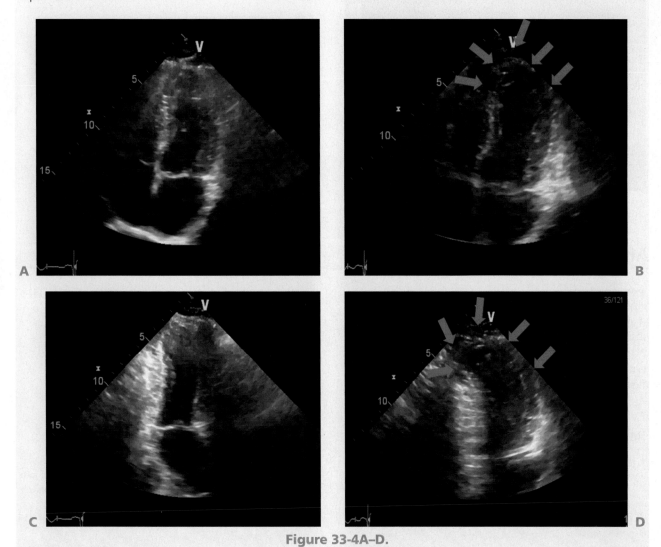

Figure 33-4A–D.

Suggested Readings

Badruddin SM, Ahmad A, Mickelson J, et al. Supine bicycle versus post-treadmill exercise echocardiography in the detection of myocardial ischemia: a randomized single-blind crossover trial. *JACC.* 1999;33:1485–1490.

Park T. Supine Bicycle Echocardiography: improved diagnostic accuracy and physiologic assessment of coronary artery disease with the incorporation of intermediate stages of exercise. *JACC.* 2007;50:1857–1863.

CASE 34

Aortic Valve Replacement after Endocarditis

*A*52-year-old man has a past history of bioprosthetic aortic valve replacement secondary to aortic valve endocarditis. He now presents to the hospital with 2 months of worsening shortness of breath and lower extremity edema. A transesophageal echocardiogram (TEE) was performed (Fig. 34-1 and Videos 34-1 to 34-4).

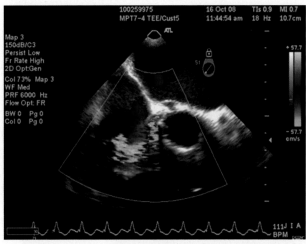

Figure 34-1.

QUESTION 1. Based on this TEE image, your diagnosis is:

A. Ventricular septal defect
B. Ruptured sinus of Valsalva
C. Gerbode defect
D. Ruptured sinus of Valsalva and Gerbode defect
E. Patent ductus arteriosus

Answers

ANSWER 1: C. The 2D echo Doppler features include a systolic, high-velocity, unidirectional flow through the lesion located between the aortic annulus and the right atrium. This is consistent with a Gerbode defect and not with a rupture of sinus of Valsalva aneurysm where the flow would be both systolic and diastolic.[1]

Reference

1. Mousavi N, Shook DC, Kilcullen N, et al. Multimodality imaging of a Gerbode defect. *Circulation.* 2012;126:e1–e2.

Suggested Reading

Cullen S, Vogel M, Deanfield JE, et al. Images in cardiovascular medicine. Rupture of aneurysm of the right sinus of Valsalva into the right ventricular outflow tract: treatment with Amplatzer atrial septal occluder. *Circulation.* 2002;105:E1–E2.

CASE 35

Weight Loss, Fatigue, Increasing Dyspnea, and Leg Edema

A 54-year-old man has suffered from weight loss and fatigue for 3 to 6 months and increasing dyspnea for 6 weeks.

Leg edema occurred over the last 4 weeks, and the patient was referred for an echocardiographic workup.

The transthoracic echocardiogram images in Videos 35-1 to 35-3 and Figures 35-1 to 35-3 were acquired.

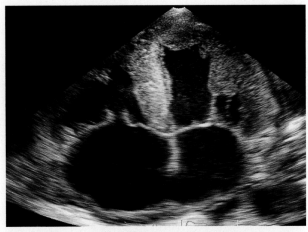

Figure 35-1. Transthoracic apical 4-chamber view.

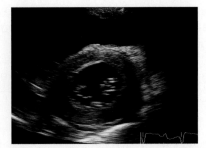

Figure 35-3. Transthoracic parasternal short-axis view.

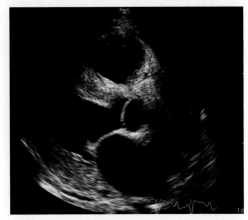

Figure 35-2. Transthoracic parasternal long-axis view.

QUESTION 1. Which is the most likely diagnosis according to these echocardiogram findings and the medical history?

    A. Hypertrophic cardiomyopathy
    B. Hypertension
    C. Cardiac amyloidosis
    D. Left ventricular noncompaction

QUESTION 2. Which diagnostic test would you suggest to confirm the diagnosis?

    A. Left heart catheterization
    B. Pericardiocentesis
    C. Myocardial biopsy
    D. Magnetic resonance imaging

Answers

ANSWER 1: C. These echocardiographic images show the typical appearance of cardiac amyloidosis in an advanced stage of the disease.

The typical features—a concentric left and right ventricular thickening, a normal left ventricular cavity size, dilated right and left atria, and a tiny pericardial effusion—can be observed in this patient.[1] The left ventricular systolic function is usually preserved up to a late stage of the disease. Diastolic dysfunction normally occurs early in cardiac amyloidosis and can be assessed by using standard and Doppler echocardiography.

A myocardial texture appearance with "granular sparkling" allows for the diagnosis of a cardiac amyloidosis with a sensitivity of 87% and specificity of 81%.[2]

ANSWER 2: C. Amyloidosis remains a tissue diagnosis; therefore, a tissue biopsy, either of an affected organ or a surrogate site (e.g., abdominal fat), is mandatory to demonstrate the disease.

Amyloid deposition is verified by classic Congo red staining or electron microscopy.

Figures 35-4 and 35-5 demonstrate the amyloid deposition by Congo red staining in an endomyocardial biopsy.

A myocardial biopsy was performed.

Once amyloidosis is diagnosed by biopsy, further clarification includes classification by the identification of the precursor protein and the assessment of disease extension (organ involvement).

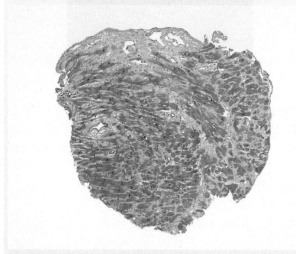

Figure 35-4. Hematoxylin-eosin staining (5×).

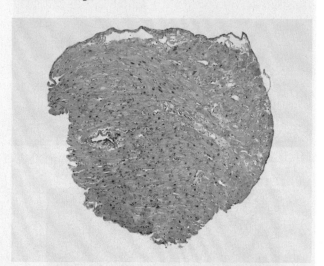

Figure 35-5. Congo red staining (5×).

References

1. Siqueira-Filho AG, Cunha CL, Tajik AJ, et al. M-Mode and two-dimensional echocardiographic features in cardiac amyloidosis. *Circulation.* 1981;63:188–196.
2. Falk RH, Plehn JF, Deering T, et al. Sensitivity and specificity of the echocardiographic features of cardiac amyloidosis. *Am J Cardiol.* 1987;59:418–422.

Suggested Readings

Cohen, AD, Comenzo RL. Systemic light-chain amyloidosis: advances in diagnosis, prognosis, and therapy. *Hematology Am Soc Hematol Educ Program.* 2010;2010:287–294.

Meier-Ewert HK, Sanchorawala V, Berk JL, Ruberg FL. Cardiac amyloidosis. Evolving approach to diagnosis and management. *Curr Treat Options Cardiovasc Med.* 2011;13(6):528–542.

Omaira H, Delgado DH. Cardiac amyloidosis: an approach to diagnosis and management. *Expert Rev Cardiovasc Ther.* 2010;8(7):1007–1013.

Diabetes, Hypertension, and Hypercholesterolemia

A 54-year-old man has diabetes, hypertension, and hypercholesterolemia. He complains of dyspnea on exertion and has limited his activities.

A stress test showed no evidence of inducible ischemia. He has a complete 2D, color, and Doppler transthoracic echocardiogram (Figs. 36-1 to 36-4 and Videos 36-1 to 36-6).

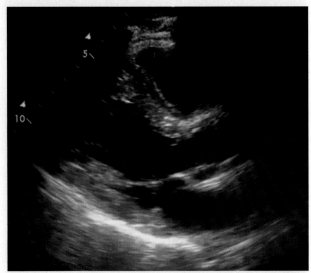

Figure 36-1.

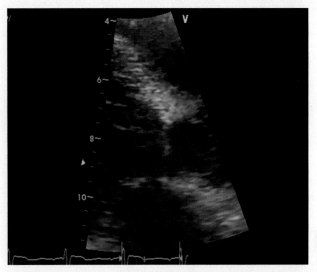

Figure 36-3.

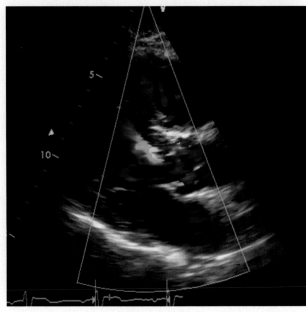

Figure 36-2.

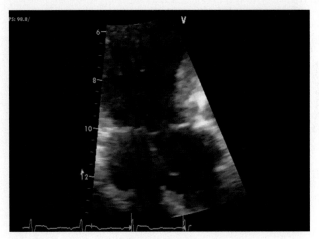

Figure 36-4.

QUESTION 1. The patient's dyspnea may be due to:

A. Severe aortic valve stenosis
B. Significant mitral regurgitation
C. Dilated cardiomyopathy
D. A subaortic membrane
E. Aortic regurgitation

Answer

ANSWER 1: D. The patient has a subaortic membrane. The images illustrate the importance of thorough interrogation of the area of the left ventricular outflow tract (LVOT) and implementing use of color Doppler. Figure 36-1 does not visualize any aortic valve disease or a membrane. Figure 36-2 demonstrates color aliasing in the LVOT, suggesting high-velocity flow. No mitral regurgitation is seen. On zoom images with the transducer slightly angulated (Figs. 36-3 and 36-4), the membrane is visualized. Additional Doppler images shown in Figures 36-5 and 36-6 confirmed a fixed (nondynamic) gradient consistent with moderate obstruction at rest. There was only minimal aortic regurgitation. A stress echocardiogram may demonstrate increased gradient correlating with the patient's symptoms during stress.

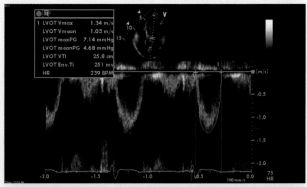

Figure 36-5. LVOT gradient proximal to the membrane – 14 mmHg.

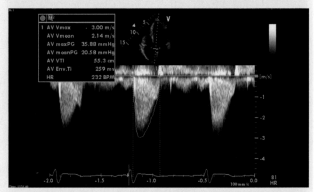

Figure 36-6. Left ventricular to aortic gradient across the membrane – 30 mmHg.

Suggested Reading

Teis A, Sheppard MN, Alpendurada F. Subaortic membrane: correlation of imaging with pathology. *Eur Heart J.* 2010;31:2822.

CASE 37

Mitral Valve Repair for Mitral Regurgitation

A 55-year-old man underwent mitral valve repair 3 months ago for symptomatic severe mitral regurgitation. He felt well until last week when he developed a recurrence of dyspnea on exertion.

On physical exam, his blood pressure is 120/60 mm Hg, pulse is 70 beats per minute and regular, neck veins are flat, and carotid pulses are normal. Lungs are clear to auscultation bilaterally. Cardiac exam reveals a well-healed midline scar, a normal S1 and S2, and no S3 gallop. There is a 2/6 holosystolic murmur at the apex that radiates to the axilla. Extremities are warm with no peripheral edema.

Echocardiography is performed to evaluate left ventricular (LV) systolic function (Figs. 37-1 to 37-4 and Videos 37-1 to 37-3).

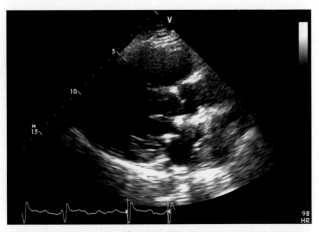

Figure 37-1.

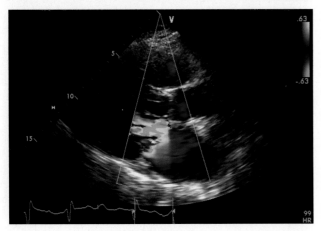

Figure 37-2.

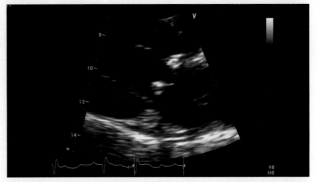

Figure 37-3.

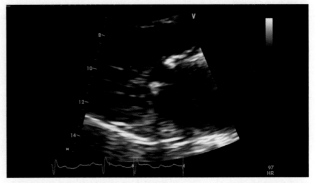

Figure 37-4.

QUESTION 1. The main abnormality on the transthoracic echocardiogram is in the region of the:

A. Aortic sinuses
B. LV outflow tract
C. Anterior mitral annulus
D. Posterior mitral annulus
E. Posterior mitral leaflet

QUESTION 2. Your recommendation would be:

A. Conservative management with repeat transthoracic echocardiogram in 1 month
B. Transesophageal echocardiography
C. Myocardial contrast echocardiography
D. Cardiac catheterization with assessment of LV pressures and ventriculography
E. Cardiac resynchronization therapy

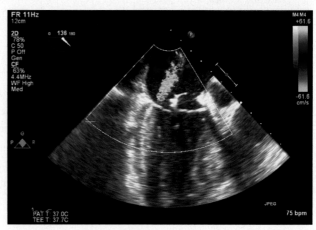

Figure 37-6.

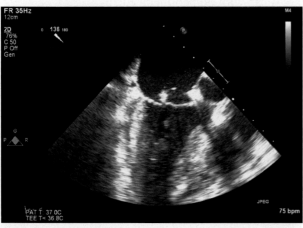

Figure 37-5.

QUESTION 3. The diagnosis is:

A. Dehiscence of the posterior aspect of the mitral annuloplasty ring
B. Normally functioning annuloplasty ring
C. Mitral annular abscess
D. Flail of the posterior leaflet
E. Flail of the anterior leaflet

Answers

ANSWER 1: D. The transthoracic echocardiogram demonstrates an abnormal space between the posterior aspect of the mitral annuloplasty ring and the posterior mitral annulus. Color Doppler shows flow behind the annuloplasty ring during diastole. The other cardiac structures described appear normal.

ANSWER 2: B. As the patient has had a change in symptoms, he should undergo transesophageal echocardiography (Figs. 37-5 and 37-6 and Videos 37-4 to 37-9) to better evaluate the degree of mitral regurgitation and function of the mitral annuloplasty ring. Blood cultures should be obtained as well, as prosthetic valve endocarditis can present insidiously.

ANSWER 3: A. There has been dehiscence of the posterior aspect of the mitral annuloplasty ring, likely secondary to undersizing of the ring for the mitral annulus. This is evident on the 2D midesophageal long-axis images and the 3D TEE video. Color Doppler shows that there is free flow around the annuloplasty ring, which is hanging freely in the left atrium.

Suggested Reading

Kronzon I, Sugeng L, Perk G, et al. Real-time 3-dimensional transesophageal echocardiography in the evaluation of postoperative mitral annuloplasty ring and prosthetic valve dehiscence. *J Am Coll Cardiol.* 2009;53:1543–1547.

CASE 38

Abrupt Onset Chest Discomfort and Abdominal Pain

A healthy 56-year-old man was in his usual state of health until he developed the abrupt onset of midsternal chest discomfort and epigastric abdominal pain. Thinking this to be indigestion, he took antacids with minimal relief of his symptoms. One day later, he developed acutely worsening shortness of breath, prompting him to call for emergency assistance.

On arrival to the emergency room, his blood pressure was 71/46 mm Hg, pulse was 115 beats per minute, and respiratory rate was 30 breaths per minute. O_2 saturation was 95% on room air. He was in moderate distress. Neck veins were distended. Lung exam demonstrated bibasilar rales. The precordial impulse was hyperdynamic, with a faint 2/6 early systolic murmur heard best in the left lower sternal border. Extremities were cool with no edema. Peripheral pulses were thread (Figs. 38-1 to 38-6 and Videos 38-1 to 38-4).

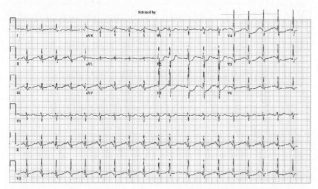

Figure 38-1. Twelve-lead electrocardiogram.

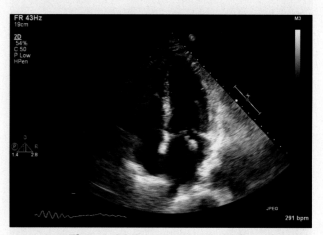

Figure 38-3. TTE, A4C: Systole.

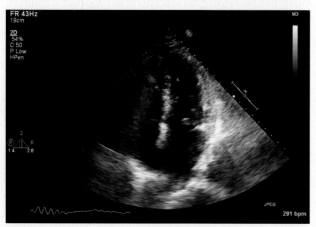

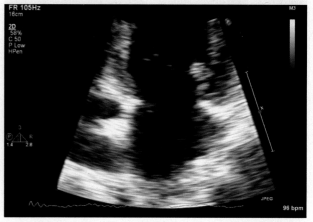

Figure 38-2. Transthoracic echocardiogram (TTE), apical four chamber (A4C): Diastole.

Figure 38-4. TTE, A4C zoomed: Diastole.

83

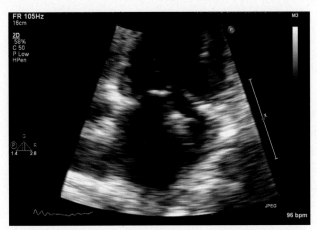

Figure 38-5. TTE, A4C zoomed: Systole.

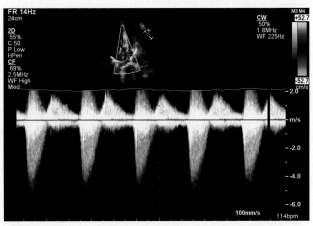

Figure 38-7. TTE continuous wave Doppler across mitral valve.

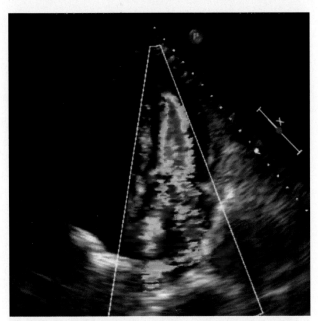

Figure 38-6. TTE, A4C color.

QUESTION 1. The most likely mechanism of mitral regurgitation in this patient is:

A. Infective endocarditis
B. Ruptured chordae tendineae with flail posterior leaflet
C. Ruptured anterolateral papillary muscle
D. Ruptured posteromedial papillary muscle
E. Malcoaptation of the posterior leaflet

QUESTION 2. The best explanation for the incomplete mitral regurgitation spectral Doppler profile in this patient is (Fig. 38-7):

A. Eccentric mitral regurgitation that moves away from the transducer
B. Rapid rise of left atrial pressures, producing a cessation of flow in late systole
C. Systolic anterior motion of the anterior mitral leaflet
D. Doppler artifact from rapid patient respiration
E. Doppler artifact from rapid heart rate

Answers

ANSWER 1: C. This patient has suffered acute rupture of the anterolateral papillary muscle with resultant acute severe mitral regurgitation. The most likely mechanism of rupture is posterior wall myocardial infarction with ischemic necrosis of the papillary muscle head. The apical four-chamber view shows the typical "meat on a stick" appearance of the necrosed papillary muscle head still attached to the mitral leaflet. Posteromedial papillary muscle rupture is more common than anterolateral papillary muscle rupture. The apical two-chamber view is the best to demonstrate which papillary muscle head is affected. The posteromedial papillary muscle is typically shown on the left (inferior wall) side, whereas the anterolateral papillary muscle is typically shown on the right (anterior wall) side. Although the findings are seen on transthoracic echocardiography in this case, transesophageal echocardiography is the best test to delineate the precise mechanism of leaflet dysfunction in a patient with acute severe mitral regurgitation.

ANSWER 2: B. The spectral Doppler profile demonstrates the "V wave cutoff sign," which is typical in acute severe mitral regurgitation. This is secondary to a midsystolic cessation of flow due to the rapid rise in left atrial pressures that occur in a patient with high regurgitant volumes and a small, noncompliant left atrium. This is also the reason that the murmur of acute severe mitral regurgitation may be faint or entirely absent.

Suggested Reading

Czarnecki A, Thakrar A, Fang T, et al. Acute severe mitral regurgitation: consideration of papillary muscle architecture. *Cardiovasc Ultrasound.* 2008;6:5.

CASE 39

Paravalvular Leak

A 57-year-old man had mechanical mitral valve replacement 3 years ago due to severe mitral regurgitation after endocarditis. Six months later, a significant paravalvular leak was verified, and a second operation was performed (St. Jude Medical mechanical valve). In the following months, he developed increasing dyspnea and leg edema. The transesophageal echocardiogram (TEE) study is shown in Videos 39-1 to 39-4 and Figures 39-1 to 39-7.

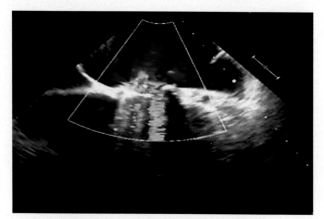

Figure 39-1. 2D TEE 18° in diastole.

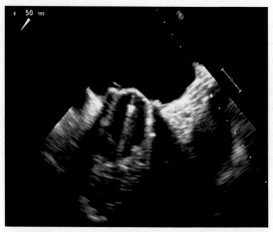

Figure 39-3. 2D TEE 50° without color Doppler.

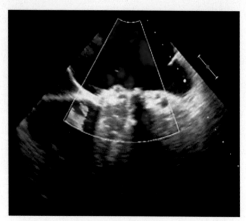

Figure 39-2. 2D TEE 18° in systole.

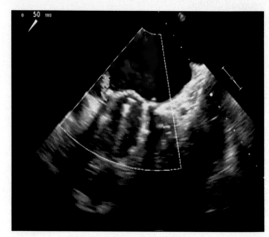

Figure 39-4. 2D TEE 50° with color Doppler.

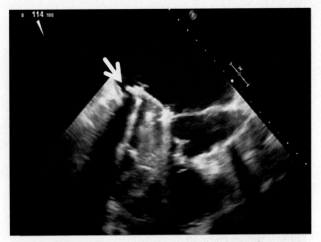

Figure 39-5. 2D TEE 114° with color Doppler.

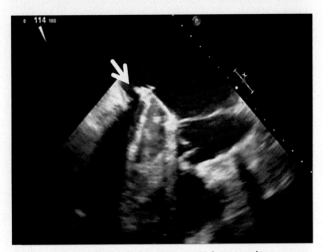

Figure 39-8. 2D TEE 114° in diastole.

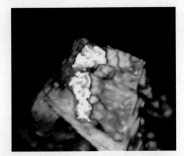

Figure 39-6. 3D full-volume aquisition with color.

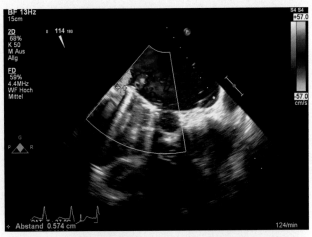

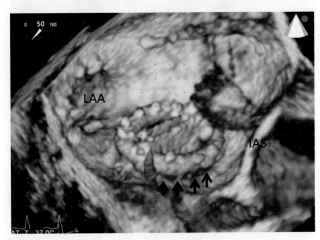

Figure 39-7.

Figure 39-9. 2D TEE 114° in systole.

QUESTION 1. Which is the correct diagnosis?

A. Paravalvular leak in anterolateral location
B. Paravalvular leak in anteromedial location
C. Paravalvular leak in posteromedial location
D. Paravalvular leak in posterolateral location

QUESTION 2. The patient underwent closure of the defect using an Amplatzer vascular plug. Two months later, the patient again complained of increasing dyspnea. The 2D TEE images (Videos 39-5 and 39-6 and Figs. 39-8 and 39-9) document the situation. Which is your diagnosis? (Select all that apply.)

A. Valve obstruction
B. Ongoing rupture of the mitral prosthetic ring
C. Infective endocarditis
D. Residual paravalvular leak
E. Device embolization

Answers

ANSWER 1: C. One potential complication after cardiac valve replacement is the development of a paravalvular leak, representing one of the most frequent causes for redo surgery.[1]

Major paravalvular leaks following surgical valve replacement are reported to occur in 1% to 5% of patients who have undergone surgical valve replacement.[2]

In this case, the defect is located posteromedially and includes approximately one-third of the circumference of the prosthetic ring.

The full-volume acquisition with color Doppler documents a broad color jet.

If a paravalvular leak is associated with symptoms due to significant regurgitation volumes or hemolysis, surgical repair is generally the preferred treatment option. However, the perioperative mortality increases with each redo procedure. After the first reoperation, a mortality rate of 13% has to be expected, increasing up to 15% after a second and 37% after a third procedure.[3]

In addition, freedom from paravalvular leak recurrence is less likely with each reoperation. Paravalvular leaks reoccur after mitral valve replacement (first redo) in 8%, in 20% after a second redo, and in 42% of patients after a third redo procedure.[4]

Due to the dimensions of the paravalvular leak in this case, surgery was considered the best treatment option, but the patient refused surgery.

Thus, a catheter-based approach to close the paravalvular leak was performed. To date, there is no standardized approach and no published best practice for this procedure. Consequently, the technical approach and results vary for each patient and even for individual lesions in the same patient.

The strategy in this case was to primarily place one occluder (Amplatzer vascular plug [AVP] III 14/5 mm, AGA Medical Corporation, Plymouth, Minnesota) and treat a residual leakage—if necessary—in a second procedure

The result after placement of an AVP III occluder is shown in Video 39-7 and Figure 39-10.

ANSWER 2: B, D. An extensive movement of the valve during the cardiac cycle can be observed ("rocking valve") in the posterior part of the ring, indicating an enlargement of the paravalvular leak.

No device can be identified posteriorly in the defect.

The 3D TEE zoom image in Figure 39-11 shows that nearly half of the circumference is ruptured, which indicates an ongoing process.

The device embolized in the distal aorta and could be snared and retrieved uneventfully.

Due to the recurrence of the paravalvar leak, the patient was sent to surgery.

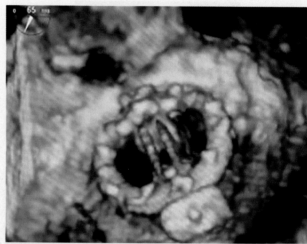

Figure 39-10. Result after placement of an AVP III occluder (14/5 mm).

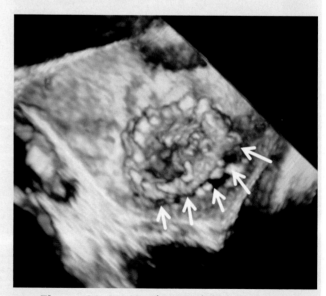

Figure 39-11. No closure device is visible.

References

1. Bernal J, Rabasa J, Gutuerrez-Garcia F, et al. The CarboMedics valve: experience with 1.049 implants. *Ann Thorac Surg.* 1998;65:137–143.
2. Pate GE, Zubaidi A, Chandavimol M, et al. Percutaneous closure of prosthetic paravalvular leaks: case series and review. *Catheter Cardiovasc Interv.* 2006;68:528–533.
3. Echevarria JR, Bernal JM, Rabasa JM, et al. Reoperation for bioprosthetic valve dysfunction: decade of clinical experience. *Eur J Cardiothorac Surg.* 1991;5:523–526.
4. ExpÓsito V, Garcia-Camarero T, Bernal JM, et al. Repeat mitral valve replacement: 30-years' experience. *Rev Esp Cardiol.* 2009;62(8):929–932.

CASE 40

Hypertension and Transient Ischemic Attack

A 57-year-old woman from El Salvador has a history of hypertension and transient ischemic attacks. She has an abnormal electrocardiogram shown in Figure 40-1.

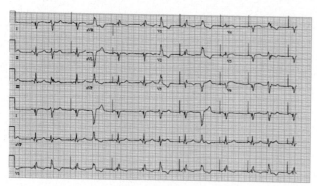

Figure 40-1.

QUESTION 1. The echocardiogram in Videos 40-1 to 40-4 shows:

A. A dilated left ventricle (LV) with basal aneurysm

B. An LV apical thrombus

C. An LV apical aneurysm

QUESTION 2. The cause of the cardiomyopathy is:

A. Ischemic; anterior infarction with development of LV apical aneurysm

B. Chagas disease

C. Noncompaction cardiomyopathy

D. Hypertensive heart disease

Answers

ANSWER 1: C The echocardiogram demonstrates a dilated LV with segmental wall motions and an apical aneurysm.

ANSWER 2: B. Chagas disease is caused by the *Triatominae* bug, *Trypanosoma cruzi*. The disease is endemic in much of Mexico and Central and South America, and more than 300,000 people with *T. cruzi* infection live in the United States.

There is a prolonged asymptomatic form. However, 20% to 30% develop chronic, often severe, symptoms. Heart rhythm abnormalities are common, and the dilated cardiomyopathy with apical aneurysm is typical for the disease. Moreover, right bundle branch block is commonly seen in patients with Chagas disease. In addition, patients may have dilatation of the esophagus and megacolon.

Suggested Readings

Acquatella H. Echocardiography in Chagas heart disease. *Circulation*. 2007;115:1124–1131.

Bern C. Evaluation and treatment of Chagas disease in the United States: a systematic review. *JAMA*. 2007;298(18):2171–2181.

CASE 41

Stress Echo for Dyspnea on Exertion

A 57-year-old woman is referred for stress echocardiogram for evaluation of dyspnea on exertion (DOE). The images in Figures 41-1 to 41-5 and Videos 41-1 to 41-2 are the pertinent findings.

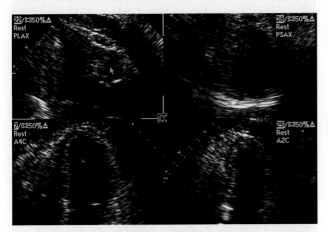

Figure 41-1.

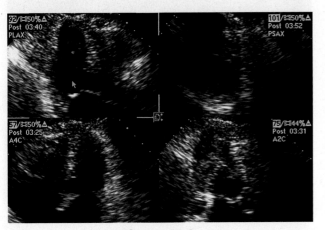

Figure 41-2.

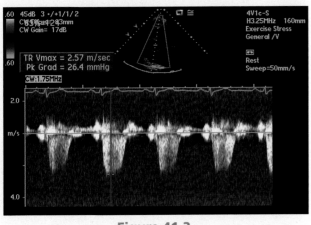

Figure 41-3.

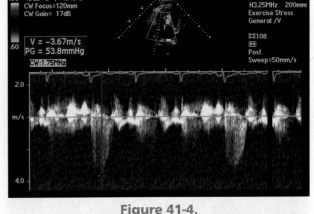

Figure 41-4.

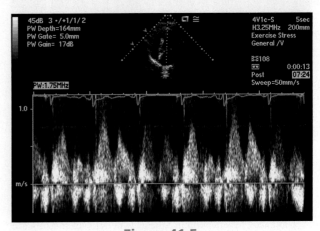

Figure 41-5.

QUESTION 1. Based on the information shown, the patient's DOE is most likely due to:

  A. Coronary artery disease
  B. Diastolic dysfunction with elevated left ventricular end diastolic (LVED) pressure
  C. Lung disease
  D. Pulmonary hypertension
  E. Lung disease and pulmonary hypertension

Answers

ANSWER 1: E. The patient has moderate-to-severe pulmonary hypertension during stress, with estimated pulmonary artery (PA) systolic pressure of 54 mm Hg plus central venous pressure. Her PA pressure was normal at rest as depicted in Figures 41-6 to 41-8. During stress, she has a normal pulmonary venous inflow pattern excluding an elevated LVED pressure as the cause of her pulmonary hypertension. There is no evidence of wall motion abnormalities at rest or during stress, making coronary artery disease much less likely.

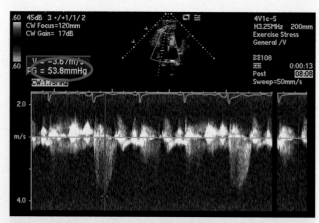

Figure 41-7. Peak RV systolic pressure.

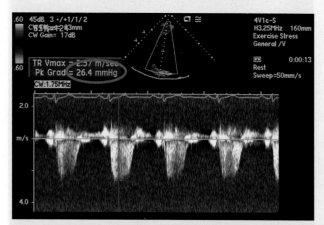

Figure 41-6. Rest right ventricular (RV) systolic pressure.

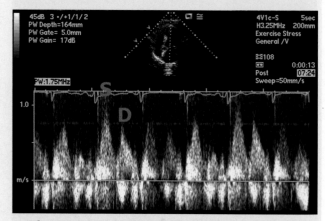

Figure 41-8. Peak pulmonary venous inflow.

Suggested Readings

Ha JW, Choi D, Park S, et al. Determinants of exercise-induced pulmonary hypertension in patients with normal left ventricular ejection fraction. *Heart.* 2009;95(6);490–494.

Singhal S, Yousuf MA, Weintraub NL, et al. Use of bicycle exercise echocardiography for unexplained exertional dyspnea. *Clin Cardiol.* 2009;32(6):302–306.

CASE 42

Rapid Atrial Fibrillation

A 61-year-old man presents to the emergency room with atrial fibrillation and a rapid ventricular response.

After anticoagulation and rate control, a transesophageal echocardiogram (TEE) is performed prior to cardioversion (Figs. 42-1 and 42-2 and Videos 42-1 and 42-2).

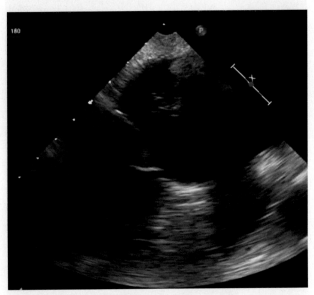

Figure 42-1.

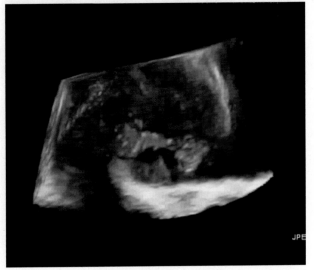

Figure 42-2.

QUESTION 1. All of the following would be appropriate *except*:

A. Continue anticoagulation

B. Perform direct current cardioversion

C. Obtain computed tomography surgery consultation

D. Order magnetic resonance imaging (MRI)

QUESTION 2. The patient underwent cardiac MRI, which showed a nonenhancing lesion. All of the following would be appropriate *except*:

A. Surgical consultation

B. Anticoagulation with clinical follow-up in 2 to 3 months

C. Anticoagulation with follow-up TEE after 4 to 6 weeks

Answers

ANSWER 1: B. All but cardioversion would be appropriate. The left atrial (LA) appendage is clearly visualized and demonstrates no thrombus (Fig. 42-3). The mass is quite large and pedunculated and appears attached to the inferior aspect of the LA wall. This is a very unusual place for the most common LA tumor, myxoma. Therefore, in a patient with atrial fibrillation, LA thrombus is still a likely diagnosis.

ANSWER 2: B. Although a nonenhancing MRI increases the likelihood that this lesion is a thrombus, myxomas do not always demonstrate enhancement, and this diagnosis cannot be entirely excluded. After 4 to 6 weeks of anticoagulation, it would be expected that a thrombus would have decreased or changed in size, whereas a myxoma would not be affected and in fact could increase in size. The risk of surgery versus the risk of embolization while waiting should be considered.

The patient was treated with heparin and then warfarin. A repeat TEE was performed 4 weeks after the first TEE and demonstrated a slight increase in the size of the mass (Fig. 42-4). This asymptomatic patient underwent surgical removal of the mass, which turned out to be an LA myxoma (Fig. 42-5).

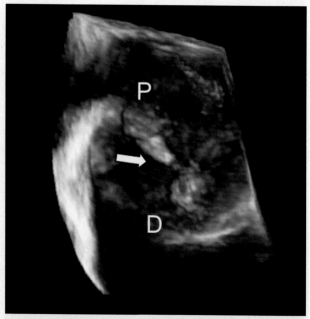

Figure 42-4. 3D echocardiography (*P*, proximal portion attached to left atrial [LA] wall; *D*, distal mobile component; *arrow*, stalk).

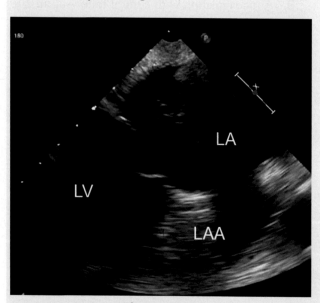

Figure 42-3.

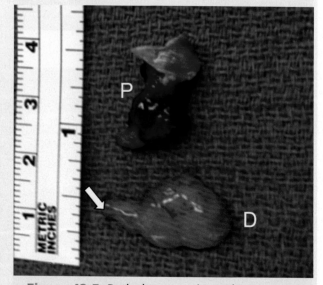

Figure 42-5. Pathology specimen (*P*, proximal portion attached to LA wall; *D*, distal mobile component; *arrow*, stalk).

Suggested Reading

Tolstrup K, Shiota T, Gurudevan S, et al. Left atrial myxomas: correlation of two-dimensional and live three-dimensional transesophageal echocardiography with the clinical and pathologic findings. *J Am Soc Echocardiogr.* 2011;24:618–624.

Resection of a Mitral Valve Tumor

*T*he patient is a 61-year-old man with a 10-year history of end-stage renal disease secondary to diabetes mellitus who is currently on hemodialysis. He was referred from an outside hospital for resection of a tumor associated with the mitral valve, which was discovered incidentally on echocardiography. He is clinically asymptomatic and denies chest pain or shortness of breath.

Physical exam reveals a chronically ill-appearing 61-year-old man in no distress. Blood pressure is 170/85 mm Hg, pulse is 88 beats per minute, and respiratory rate is 20 breaths per minute. Lungs are clear to auscultation bilaterally. Chest shows scars on the anterior chest wall from previous vascular access sites. Cardiac exam reveals a nondisplaced point of maximum impulse with normal S1 and S2 and an S4 gallop. There is a faint 2/6 holosystolic murmur in the left lower sternal border that does not radiate. See Videos 43-1 to 43-5.

QUESTION 1. The most likely diagnosis is:
A. Mitral valve endocarditis with mitral annular abscess
B. Caseous calcification of the mitral valve annulus
C. Left atrial myxoma
D. Mitral valve papillary fibroelastoma
E. Mitral valve prolapse

QUESTION 2. The best management option for this patient would be:
A. Mitral valve replacement
B. Mitral valve repair
C. Mitral and aortic valve replacement
D. Aortic valve replacement
E. No cardiac surgery is necessary at this time

Answers

ANSWER 1: B. The transthoracic echocardiogram demonstrates evidence of a large calcific mass along the posterior aspect of the mitral annulus. There is central echolucency, consistent with the diagnosis of caseous calcification of the mitral annulus. There is normal function of the mitral valve with mild mitral regurgitation and very mild mitral stenosis.

ANSWER 2: E. Caseous calcification of the mitral annulus (CCMA) is a rare variant of mitral annular calcification (MAC), constituting about 0.63% of all MAC cases. Although CCMA is usually a benign, asymptomatic condition, it is often misconstrued as a cardiac tumor, a thrombus, or an abscess, which leads to unnecessary investigations and interventions. In the absence of significant mitral stenosis or mitral regurgitation, surgical intervention is not indicated in patients with caseous calcification of the mitral annulus. The internal material is caseous and putty-like material and is surrounded by a calcified envelope. Microscopic examination shows this material to be amorphous, acellular, basophilic, and calcific, with a mild chronic inflammatory reaction manifested mainly by macrophages.

Suggested Reading

Arora H, Madan P, Simpson L, et al. Caseous calcification of the mitral annulus. *Tex Heart Inst J.* 2008;35(2):211–213.

Coronary Artery Bypass Graft and Aortic Valve Replacement

A 61-year-old man with a history of coronary artery bypass grafting and aortic valve replacement presents with worsening fatigue and dyspnea on exertion for the past 3 months. About 1 month ago, he noted a twinge of chest pain and, following this, his symptoms became much worse. He denies fever, chills, or rigors. On presentation to the emergency room, he is found to be in florid hypoxic respiratory failure and is intubated.

On physical exam, blood pressure is 161/45 mm Hg, pulse is 110 beats per minute and regular, neck veins are distended, and carotid pulses are brisk. Lungs are clear to auscultation bilaterally. Cardiac exam reveals a well-healed midline scar, a normal S1 and S2 with no S3 or S4 gallops. There is a 3/6 continuous murmur in the left upper sternal border that is nonradiating. Extremities are cool with no peripheral edema.

The patient undergoes a transesophageal echocardiogram (TEE) shown in Videos 44-1 to 44-4.

QUESTION 1. The transesophageal echocardiogram shows a rupture of the:

A. Posterior mitral leaflet
B. Right coronary cusp
C. Posteromedial papillary muscle
D. Anterolateral papillary muscle
E. Mitral intervalvular fibrosa

QUESTION 2. The continuous murmur likely results from flow between the:

A. Aorta and right atrium (RA)
B. Aorta and left atrium (LA)
C. Left ventricle (LV) and RA
D. LV and right ventricle
E. None of the options

Answers

ANSWER 1: E. The TEE demonstrates a perforation through the mitral intravalvular fibrosa and the aortic sinus consistent with an aortic root abscess. This is seen on the 2D and 3D TEE color Doppler.

ANSWER 2: B. As the pressure in the aorta is higher in the LA throughout systole and diastole, there is continuous flow from the aorta to the LA, which results in a continuous murmur.

Suggested Reading

Leung DY, Cranney GB, Hopkins AP, et al. Role of transoesophageal echocardiography in the diagnosis and management of aortic root abscess. *Br Heart J.* 1994;72:175–181.

CASE 45

Worsening Abdominal Bloating

A 61-year-old retired physician presents with a 6-month history of worsening midepigastric bloating sensation associated with fatigue, diarrhea, and lower extremity edema. He has occasional episodes of heat intolerance and has had a 15-lb weight loss.

Physical examination reveals a thin, fatigued, chronically ill-appearing 61-year-old man in no acute distress. Blood pressure is 110/60 mm Hg, pulse is 90 beats per minute, and respiratory rate is 18 breaths per minute. Neck veins are elevated to the level of the jaw. Lungs are clear to auscultation. There is a right parasternal lift and a palpable right ventricular heave. There is a normal S1 and S2 with a 3/6 holosystolic murmur heard best in the left lower sternal border. Abdomen is distended with evidence of 3 mm of shifting dullness and a palpable fluid wave. There is 3+ pitting edema extending to the midthigh (Fig. 45-1 and Videos 45-1 to 45-7).

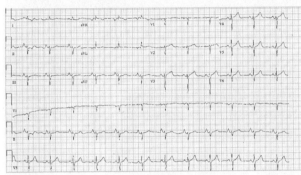

Figure 45-1.

QUESTION 1. The primary valvular lesions are:

- A. Mitral and aortic regurgitation
- B. Mitral regurgitation only
- C. Tricuspid regurgitation only
- D. Tricuspid and pulmonary regurgitation
- E. Aortic, mitral, and tricuspid regurgitation

QUESTION 2. The most likely cause of this patient's valvular heart disease is:

- A. Hyperthyroidism
- B. Rheumatic heart disease
- C. Carcinoid heart disease
- D. Infective endocarditis
- E. Radiation valvulitis

Answers

ANSWER 1: D. The transthoracic echocardiogram images demonstrate retraction and fibrosis of the tricuspid and pulmonary valves. There is evidence of severe tricuspid regurgitation and severe pulmonary regurgitation. The left-sided valves are normal in appearance and demonstrate normal function.

ANSWER 2: C. The appearance of the tricuspid and pulmonary valves are classic for carcinoid heart disease. Carcinoid tumor is a neuroendocrine tumor that occurs in the gastrointestinal tract and lungs. It has a propensity to metastasize to the liver and when it does so, it releases large amounts of serotonin (5-hydroxyindole-acetic acid), causing fibrosis of the valves on the right side of the heart. The serotonin is metabolized in the lungs, so left-sided valvular heart disease is usually not seen unless there is an associated patent foramen ovale.

Suggested Reading

Nalawadi SS, Siegel RJ, Wolin E, et al. Morphologic features of carcinoid heart disease as assessed by three-dimensional transesophageal echocardiography. *Echocardiography*. 2010;27(9):1098–1105.

Pulmonary Edema and End-Stage Renal Disease

A 61-year-old woman with New York Heart Association classification class III heart failure has a history of pulmonary edema and end-stage renal disease.

She was found to have aortic valve stenosis and underwent aortic valve replacement. Postoperatively, she had fevers and pulmonary congestion.

Please see the transthoracic echocardiogram (TTE) images in Figures 46-1 to 46-5 and Videos 46-1 to 46-3.

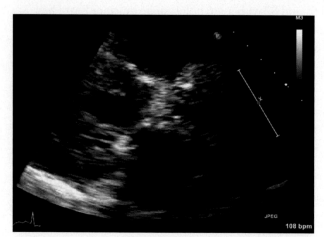

Figure 46-1.

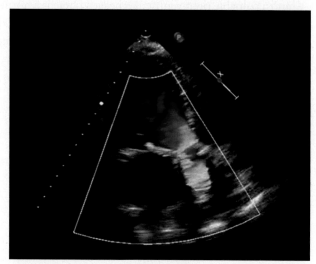

Figure 46-3.

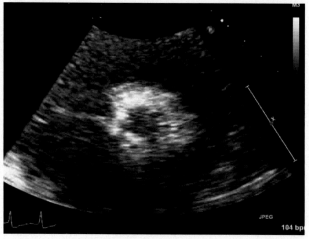

Figure 46-2.

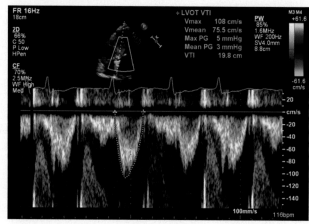

Figure 46-4.

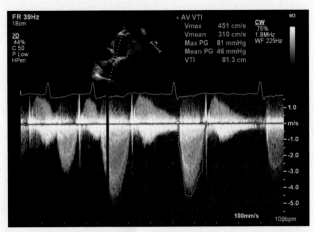

Figure 46-5.

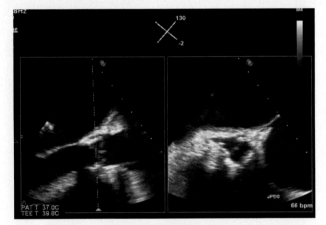

Figure 46-6.

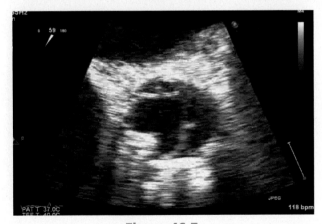

Figure 46-7.

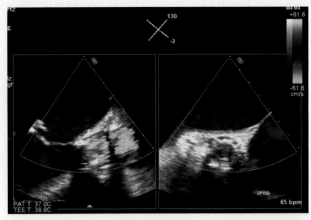

Figure 46-8.

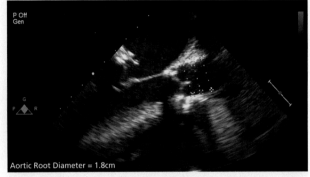

Figure 46-9.

QUESTION 1. The postoperative TTE to evaluate left ventricular (LV) function demonstrates findings consistent with which of the following (select all that apply)?

    A. A bioprosthetic aortic valve

    B. A mechanical prosthetic aortic valve

    C. An aortic valve vegetation

    D. Prosthetic aortic valve stenosis

QUESTION 2. The postoperative transesophageal echocardiogram (TEE) done to exclude a vegetation and further evaluate the cause of the elevated aortic valve gradient (Figs. 46-6 to 46-11 and Videos 46-4 to 46-6) demonstrates which of the following (select all that apply)?

    A. A bioprosthetic aortic valve, which opens normally

    B. A stenotic bioprosthetic aortic valve

    C. An aortic valve vegetation

    D. Pseudoaortic stenosis

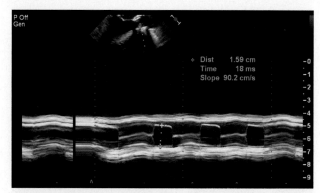

Figure 46-10.

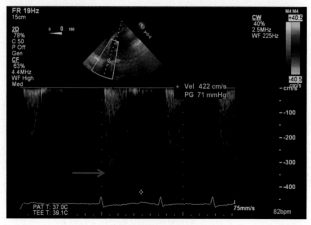

Figure 46-11.

QUESTION 3. The postoperative TEE was useful in showing that the aortic valve gradient is due to which of the following (select all that apply)?

A. Pseudoaortic stenosis
B. Abnormal pressure recovery
C. A small aortic root
D. A supravalvar membrane

Answers

ANSWER 1: A, D. The TTE demonstrates findings consistent with both a bioprosthetic aortic valve and prosthetic aortic valve stenosis.

ANSWER 2: A, D. The postoperative TEE demonstrates both a bioprosthetic aortic valve, which opens normally, and pseudoaortic stenosis.

ANSWER 3: A, B, C. The postoperative TEE was useful in showing that the aortic valve gradient is due to pseudoaortic stenosis, abnormal pressure recovery, and a small aortic root.

SUBSEQUENT FINDINGS

Pressure recovery

- Clinically relevant if aortic root diameter < 3 cm
- Convergence of flow through a stenotic AV valve to the vena contracta (VC) convert potential energy to kinetic energy → drop in the pressure at the VC.
- As flow diverges and slows again distal to the VC there is reconversion of kinetic energy to potential energy with recovery of a proportion of the pressure lost from the LVOT to the VC.
- As Doppler detect peak velocity at the VC, the transvalvular pressure drop by Doppler is > calculated from catheterization measurements in the LVOT and aortic root distal to the VC → pressure recovery Doppler underestimates aortic valve area and thus overestimates AS severity compared to catheter based methods.

Pressure recovery can be calculated:

$$4v^2 \times 2AVA/Aa \times [1 - (AVA/Aa)]$$
V = maximum Doppler transvalvular velocity
AVA = by the continuity equation
Aa = is the ascending aortic area

Pressure recovery adjusted AVAI [cm^2/m^2]
$$AVA \times Aa/(Aa - AVA)/m^2)$$

Severe aortic stenosis (AS) defined as AVAI ≤ 0.6 cm^2/m^2.

If we use these data, we can calculate the true aortic valve area in our patient with a very small aortic root:

BSA:	1.56 m^2
Ao diameter:	~2 cm = 3.14 cm^2
AVA:	0.69 cm^2
	− [(1.9^2 × 0.785) × 19.8] / 81
AVAI:	0.44 cm^2/m^2
Pressure recovery:	~27 mm Hg
Corrected AVAI:	~1.4 cm^2/m^2

Thus, as shown below (Table 46-1), our patient has a normal bioprosthetic aortic valve area when pressure recovery is considered.

AV mean G	46.0 mm Hg	→	19 mm Hg
AVA:	0.69 cm^2	→	1.28 cm^2

TABLE 46-1.

Valve	Size	Peak gradient (mm Hg)	Mean gradient (mm Hg)	Effective orifice area (cm^2)
Mitroflow *Stented bovine pericardial*	19	18.6 ± 5.3	13.1 ± 3.33	1.1 ± 0.2

Suggested Reading

Niederberger J, Schima H, Maurer G, et al. Importance of pressure recovery for the assessment of aortic stenosis by Doppler ultrasound. Role of aortic size, aortic valve area, and direction of the stenotic jet in vitro. *Circulation.* 1996;94:1934–1940.

CASE 47

Mitral Valve Replacement and Hypotension

*T*he patient is a 62-year-old man who underwent mitral valve replacement. Six hours after returning to the intensive care unit, he develops hypotension with a systolic blood pressure (BP) of 70 mm Hg and a heart rate of 120 beats per minute. Normal saline is given (500 mL), the systolic BP on norepinephrine is 75 mm Hg, and the central venous pressure is 20 mm Hg.

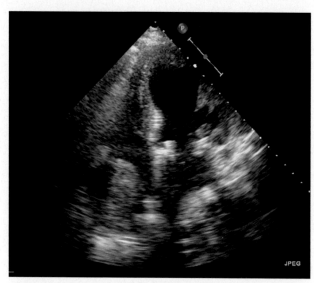

Figure 47-1.

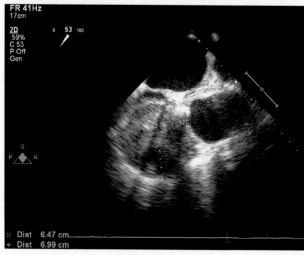

Figure 47-2.

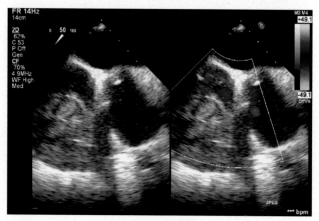

Figure 47-3.

QUESTION 1. This transthoracic echocardiogram (Fig. 47-1 and Video 47-1) shows (select all that apply):

    A. Bioprosthetic mitral valve

    B. An underfilled right ventricle (RV)

    C. A clot within the right atrium

    D. A clot compressing the right atrium

QUESTION 2. You recommend:

    A. Giving more intravenous fluids

    B. Taking the patient back to the operating room (OR) to remove the clot

QUESTION 3. The cardiac surgeon wants a transesophageal echocardiogram (TEE) to better evaluate the patient before going back to the OR. The TEE (Figs. 47-2 and 47-3 and Videos 47-2 and 47-3) shows (select all that apply):

    A. A tumor within the left atrium

    B. A clot within the right atrium

    C. A clot compressing the right atrium

    D. None of the options

Answers

ANSWER 1: A, B, D. The transthoracic echocardiogram shows bioprosthetic mitral valve, an underfilled RV, and a clot compressing the right atrium.

ANSWER 2: B. Recommend taking the patient back to the OR to remove the clot.

ANSWER 3: B, C. Conventional transthoracic 2D echocardiography is frequently suboptimal immediately after open heart surgery (due to limited windows) to identify pericardial effusion, localized RV or right atrial compression, and blood or an organized clot. TEE is often critical in making the diagnosis of postcardiac surgery tamponade because TTE is technically limited, and the site of tamponade can be localized so that it can only be detected by TEE.

Figure 47-4 shows the clot that was found compressing the right atrium at the time of re-operation.

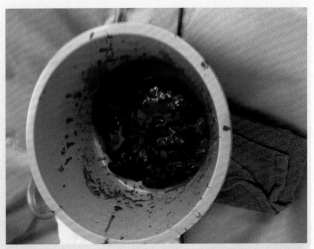

Figure 47-4.

Suggested Readings

Chuttani K, Tischler MD, Pandian NG, et al. Diagnosis of cardiac tamponade after cardiac surgery: relative value of clinical, echocardiographic, and hemodynamic signs. *Am Heart J.* 1994;127:913–918.

Kochar GS, Jacobs LE, Kotler MN. Right atrial compression in postoperative cardiac patients: detection by transesophageal echocardiography. *J Am Coll Cardiol.* 1990;16:511–516.

CASE 48

Degenerative Mitral Regurgitation

A 63-year-old woman with dyspnea on exertion is diagnosed with degenerative mitral regurgitation due to a myxomatous mitral valve. She is referred for mitral valve surgery, and her intraoperative transesophageal echocardiogram (TEE) images are shown in Videos 48-1 to 48-6 and Figures 48-1 to 48-6.

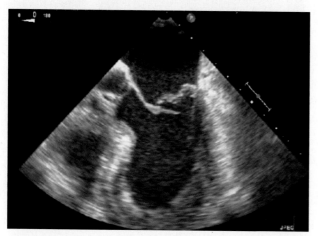

Figure 48-1.

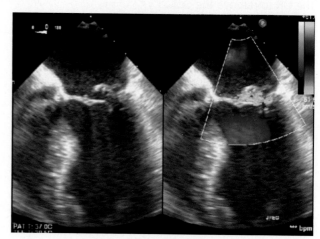

Figure 48-3.

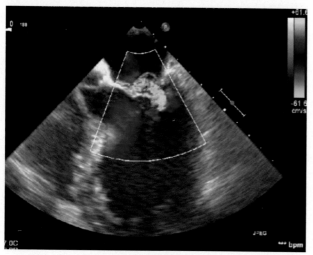

Figure 48-2.

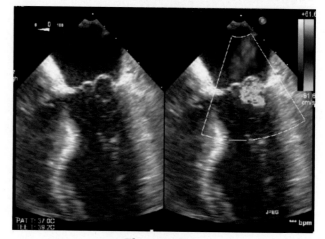

Figure 48-4.

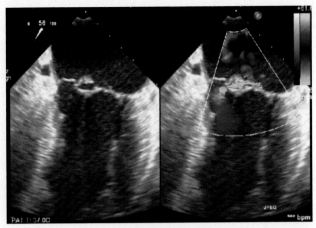

Figure 48-5.

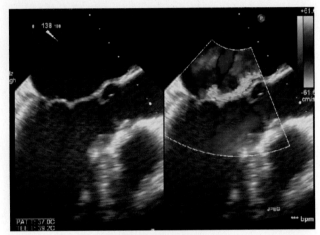

Figure 48-6.

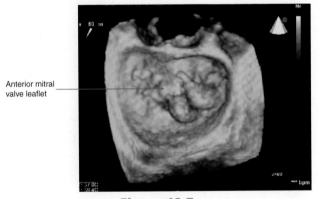

Anterior mitral
valve leaflet

Figure 48-7.

QUESTION 1. Which scallop(s) of the mitral valve are prolapsed and/or flail?

A. P1 and P2

B. P2 and P3

C. P2 only

D. Cannot be determined on the basis of the images provided—additional imaging is recommended

E. A1 and P3

QUESTION 2. With the additional information afforded by a 3D TEE (Fig. 48-7 and Video 48-7), which scallop(s) of the mitral valve are prolapsed and/or flail?

A. P1 and P2

B. P2 and P3

C. P2 only

D. A2 only

E. A1 and P3

Answers

ANSWER 1: D. TEE Videos 48-1 and 48-2 suggest flail of the P1 and possibly P2 scallops of the posterior mitral leaflets. TEE Video 48-4 does not show a flail of the P2 or P3 scallops of the posterior mitral leaflet. Video 48-5, the intercommissural view, shows prolapse and flail of P2 and P3. The data from 2D TEE are thus contradictory. Additional imaging with a 3D TEE is performed (Fig. 48-7 and Video 48-7).

ANSWER 2: B. 3D TEE and direct visualization of the valve during cardiac surgery (Video 48-8) show that the P2 (middle) and P3 (medial) scallops are prolapsed and flail. The patient underwent successful mitral valve repair with placement of an annuloplasty ring preoperatively or intraoperatively. 3D TEE is very helpful prior to mitral valve repair as it enables the echocardiographer to visualize the specific mechanism of mitral regurgitation and helps the surgeon to identify the culprit scallop(s).

Suggested Reading

Chandra S, Salgo IS, Sugeng L, et al. Characterization of degenerative mitral valve disease using morphologic analysis of real-time three-dimensional echocardiographic images: objective insight into complexity and planning of mitral valve repair. *Circ Cardiovasc Imaging.* 2011;4:24–32.

CASE 49

Bioprosthetic Mitral Valve Replacement

*A*65-year-old man had a bioprosthetic mitral valve (MV) replacement 6 years ago. He now presents with worsening congestive heart failure (CHF). A transesophageal echocardiogram is done to evaluate the cause of the CHF and the bioprosthetic MV function and morphology (Videos 49-1 and 49-2).

QUESTION 1. The cause of the CHF is:

A. Severe mitral regurgitation (MR)
B. Impaired left ventricular function
C. Degeneration of the bioprosthetic MV
D. Paraprosthetic MR

QUESTION 2. See Videos 49-1 to 49-3. Is this leak amenable to catheter closure?

A. Yes
B. No

QUESTION 3. See Videos 49-4 and 49-5. The catheter is across:

A. The bioprosthetic MV orifice
B. The paravalvular leak

QUESTION 4. See Videos 49-6 to 49-8. The guide catheter is across:

A. The paravalvular leak
B. The valve orifice

Answers

ANSWER 1: D. In addition, the patient has hemolysis, which is common in patients with paraprosthetic MR.

ANSWER 2: A. This defect should be amenable to percutaneous closure because the defect does not exceed 33% of the circumference of the prosthetic valve.

ANSWER 3: A. With 3D imaging, it is clear that the catheter is across the valve.

ANSWER 4: A. With 3D imaging, it is clear that the catheter is across the paravalvular leak.

SUBSEQUENT FINDINGS
See in Videos 49-9 and 49-10 the Amplatzer device closing the perivalvular leak. There is a good result post-deployment (Videos 49-11 to 49-13 and Fig. 49-1).

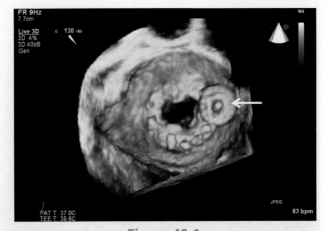

Figure 49-1.

Suggested Reading

Ruiz CE. Clinical outcomes in patients undergoing percutaneous closure of periprosthetic paravalvular leaks. *Am J Cardiol.* 2011;58:2210–2217.

CASE 50

Cirrhosis of the Liver and Myocardial Infarction

A 65-year-old man from Uruguay has a history of cirrhosis of the liver and a prior myocardial infarction. The echocardiogram (Videos 50-1 to 50-5) is done as part of a pre-liver transplant screening evaluation.

QUESTION 1. The echocardiogram findings are consistent with:

- A. Chagas disease
- B. Inferolateral wall pseudoaneurysm
- C. A true inferolateral wall aneurysm
- D. Pseudodyskinesis of the inferolateral wall

QUESTION 2. You recommend:

- A. Urgent surgery
- B. Medical management
- C. Another test

Answers

ANSWER 1: C. True aneurysms generally have a wide mouth, whereas pseudoaneurysms generally have a narrow neck, as shown in Figure 50-1.

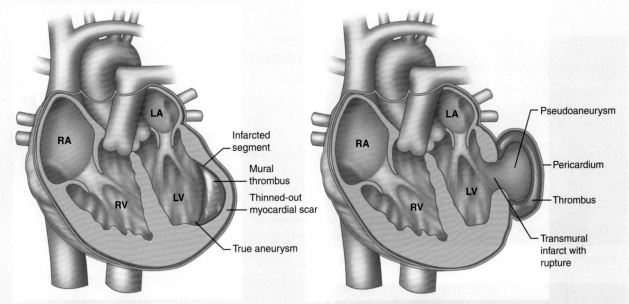

True aneurysm

1. Wide base
2. Walls composed of myocardium
3. Low risk of rupture

Pseudoaneurysm

1. Narrow base
2. Walls composed of thrombus and pericardium
3. High risk of rupture

Figure 50-1.

ANSWER 2: B. Medical management is the appropriate choice. Another test is okay if you are not sure. If you are uncertain about the diagnosis, additional testing could include a contrast echocardiogram, computed tomography, or magnetic resonance imaging scan with contrast.

If you are concerned about Chagas disease, a blood test for detecting *Trypanosoma cruzi*, the anti–*T. cruzi* assay, could be ordered.

This patient died secondary to his liver disease. As seen in Figure 50-2, at autopsy, the pathologic findings confirmed an inferolateral left ventricular aneurysm. The neck of the aneurysm is wide, and the myocardium, although thin, extends around the perimeter of the aneurysm.

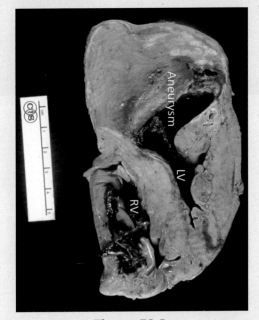

Figure 50-2.

Suggested Reading

Centers for Disease Control and Prevention. Parasites–American trypanosomiasis (also known as Chagas disease). http://www.cdc.gov/parasites/chagas/health_professionals/dx.html.

CASE 51

Obesity and Dyspnea on Exertion

A 65-year-old obese woman gets admitted to the hospital with complaints of shortness of breath and dyspnea on exertion.

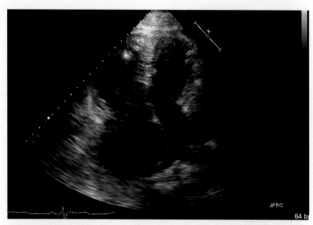

Figure 51-1. Transthoracic four-chamber view.

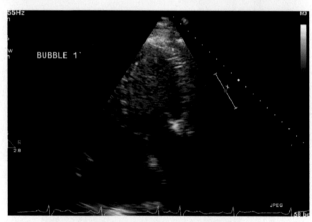

Figure 51-2. Saline contrast study.

QUESTION 1. Figures 51-1 and 51-2 and Videos 51-1 and 51-2 show:

  A. An enlarged left ventricle and a right-to-left shunt

  B. An enlarged right ventricle and a left-to-right shunt

  C. An enlarged right atrium and right ventricle and a right-to-left shunt

QUESTION 2. The next best step would be:

  A. A right and left heart catheterization

  B. A transesophageal echocardiogram (TEE)

  C. Placement of transcatheter atrial septal occluder device

  D. A right heart catheterization with measurement of saturations

  E. Start medical treatment of pulmonary hypertension

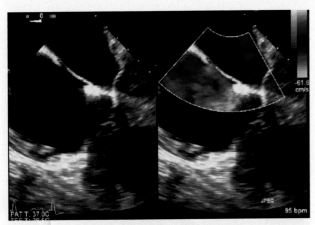

Figure 51-3.

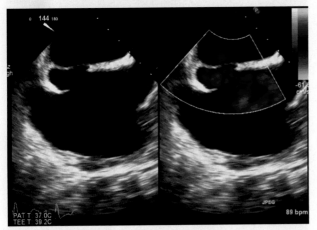

Figure 51-4.

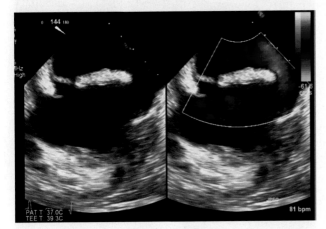

Figure 51-5.

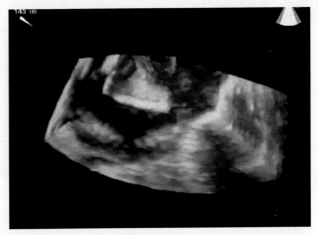

Figure 51-6.

QUESTION 3. Figures 51-3 to 51-6 and Videos 51-3 to 51-5 demonstrate:

    A. A secundum atrial septal defect (ASD)

    B. A patent foramen ovale

    C. A superior sinus venous defect

    D. An inferior sinus venous defect

Answers

ANSWER 1: C. The transthoracic images are of fair quality due to the patient's body habits. The first image shows a markedly enlarged right heart with right ventricular hypertrophy and the interatrial septum bulging to the right, consistent with both the patient's pulmonary hypertension and elevated right atrial pressure. The second image shows opacification of the left ventricle with saline contrast, confirming a large right-to-left shunt. The opacification was almost immediate, but the exact site of the shunt was not visualized on this study.

ANSWER 2: B. A TEE to identify the anatomy and site of the shunt would be a very reasonable first step. If a secundum atrial defect, which is the most common ASD, is detected then the TEE would help assess if the patient would be a candidate for a septal occluder device. There is no indication for a left heart catheterization. A right heart catheterization with saturations may still be indicated to evaluate the physiology of the shunt and evaluate pulmonary vascular resistance but would not clarify if the patient would be a candidate for percutaneous closure of an ASD. Correction of the intracardiac defect may be indicated rather than medical treatment of the pulmonary hypertension.

ANSWER 3: C. The images demonstrate a communication between the rupv and the svc, consistent with a superior sinus venous defect (Figs. 51-7 to 51-10). As sinus venous defects are not amenable to percutaneous device closure, the patient was referred for surgery. (*, intact interatrial septum; rupv, right upper pulmonary vein; svc, superior vena cava.)

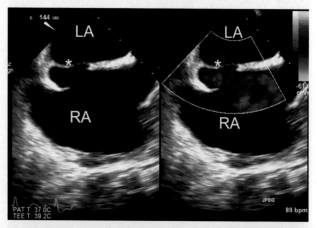

Figure 51-8.

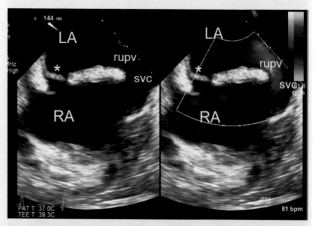

Figure 51-9.

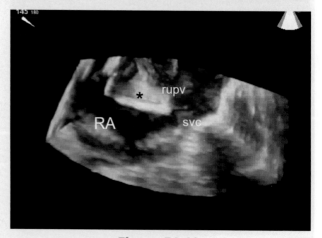

Figure 51-10.

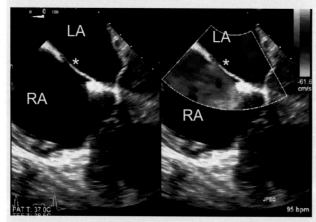

Figure 51-7.

Suggested Reading

Ahn J, Park SH, Kim D, et al. Role of echocardiography in sinus venous atrial septal defect combined with systemic and pulmonary vascular disease. *J Cardiovasc Ultrasound.* 2012;20:49–51.

CASE 52

Upper Respiratory Complaints

A 65-year-old woman presents to her primary care physician with upper respiratory complaints. She later develops progressively worsening dyspnea on exertion and cough.

She is treated with antibiotics with limited resolution of her symptoms.

Transthoracic echocardiography (TTE) is performed. Figures 52-1 and 52-2 and Videos 52-1 and 52-2 show the parasternal long axis and apical four-chamber views, and no abnormalities were seen.

Two months later, the patient is hospitalized after presenting to her ophthalmologist, complaining of loss of vision in her right eye. Retinal examination reveals evidence of an embolus to the right eye.

Brain magnetic resonance imaging reveals evidence of cerebral infarction localized to the caudate nucleus and both cerebellar hemispheres.

TTE is repeated; Figure 52-3 and Video 52-3 show apical four-chamber view.

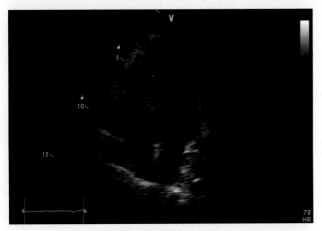

Figure 52-1.

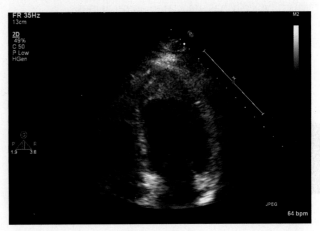

Figure 52-3.

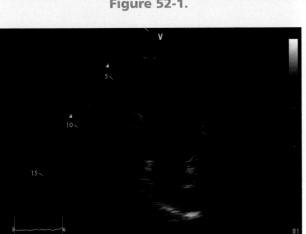

Figure 52-2.

QUESTION 1. Which diagnostic test or procedure should be initially performed to confirm the diagnosis?

- A. Left ventricular endomyocardial biopsy
- B. Left heart catheterization and coronary angiography
- C. Myocardial perfusion single-photon emission computed tomography
- D. Complete blood count with differential
- E. Myocardial contrast echocardiography

Answers

ANSWER 1: D. This patient has Loeffler disease, one of a group of hypereosinophilic syndromes with mutations in genes encoding for tyrosine kinase receptor, platelet-derived growth factor receptors. Heart damage evolves through three stages: (1) an acute necrotic stage, (2) an intermediate stage characterized by thrombus formation along the damaged endocardium, and (3) a fibrotic stage. Diagnosis should be confirmed initially with complete blood count with differential, which demonstrates significant eosinophilia.

The echocardiogram in Loeffler disease demonstrates filling of the left ventricular apex with thrombotic material with preserved contraction of the apical myocardial segments. This is in contrast to apical mural thrombus, which typically has associated apical akinesis.

Video 52-4 demonstrates an apical four-chamber view with microbubble contrast, which better illustrates the region of thrombotic material in the left ventricular apex.

Endomyocardial biopsy confirms diagnosis of Loeffler endomyocardial fibrosis (Fig. 52-4).

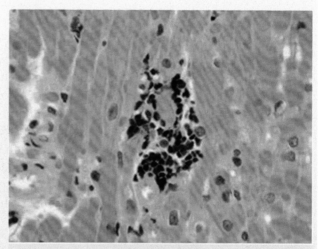

Figure 52-4.

Suggested Reading

Chang SA, Kim HK, Park EA, et al. Images in cardiovascular medicine. Loeffler endocarditis mimicking apical hypertrophic cardiomyopathy. *Circulation.* 2009;120:82–85.

CASE 53

Congestive Heart Failure with a Biventricular Pacemaker

A 65-year-old woman with congestive heart failure and a biventricular pacemaker had two hospitalizations for heart failure in the past 6 months. She has a midpeaking systolic murmur heard best at the base. She has severe emphysema and is very frail.

She is referred for evaluation of aortic stenosis and in consideration for percutaneous aortic valve replacement (Figs. 53-1 and 53-2 and Video 53-1).

After echocardiogram contrast, the peak velocity increased from 296 cm per second to 331 cm per second, whereas the mean gradient increased from 23 to 24 mm Hg, and the aortic valve area calculates to 0.68 cm² (Fig. 53-3).

In order to qualify for the percutaneous aortic valve, the peak velocity needs to be ≥ 4 m per second, and the mean aortic valve gradient needs to be ≥ 40 mm Hg.

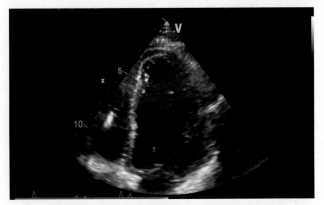

Figure 53-1.

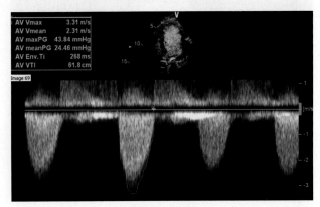

Figure 53-3.

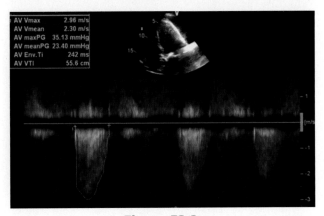

Figure 53-2.

QUESTION 1. Based on the clinical history and the data shown in Figures 53-1 to 53-3 and Video 53-1:

  A. You decide the patient's primary problem is left ventricular dysfunction and not the aortic stenosis

  B. You refer the patient to the cardiac surgery for the aortic valve replacement

  C. You refer the patient for dobutamine stress echocardiography to further evaluate the low-gradient aortic stenosis

  D. You refer the patient for chelation therapy to decalcify the aortic valve

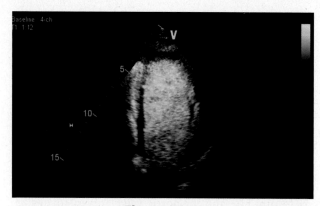

Figure 53-4.

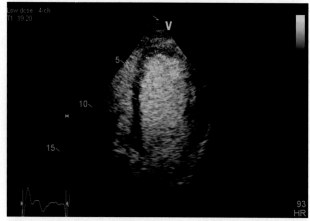

Figure 53-5.

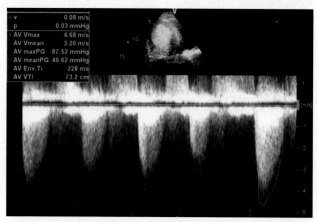

Figure 53-6. Dobutamine study (20 mcg). Peak and mean gradients increased, and aortic valve area decreased from 0.68 to 0.57 cm². Peak velocity, 468 cm per second; peak gradient, 87 mm Hg; mean gradient, 49 mm Hg; and aortic valve area, 0.57 cm².

QUESTION 2. Based on the echo Doppler findings on Figures 53-4 to 53-6 and Videos 53-2 and 53-3, does this patient have severe aortic stenosis?

    A. Yes
    B. No

Answers

ANSWER 1: C. You refer the patient for dobutamine stress echocardiography to further evaluate the low-gradient aortic stenosis.

    In evaluating patients with aortic stenosis, whether it's a discrepancy between gradients and cusp excursion, dobutamine stress echo (dose 5 to 20 mcg) has been shown to be of value to identify patients with true aortic stenosis and differentiate from pseudoaortic stenosis, which can be seen in low output syndrome.

ANSWER 2: A. During dobutamine, the peak and mean aortic valve gradients rose, and the valve area fell. These findings are indicative of severe aortic stenosis.

    This patient will now qualify for percutaneous aortic valve replacement.

Suggested Reading

Lange RA, Hillis LD. Dobutamine stress echocardiography in patients with low-gradient aortic stenosis. *Circulation.* 2006; 113:1718–1720.

CASE 54

Percutaneous Coronary Intervention and Stenting

A 65-year-old woman with a history of coronary artery disease, prior coronary artery bypass graft 13 years ago, and coronary angioplasty with stent placement twice in the last 10 years developed shortness of breath and was found to have severe mitral regurgitation on echocardiography. She subsequently had mitral valve repair but after surgery had persistent shortness of breath.

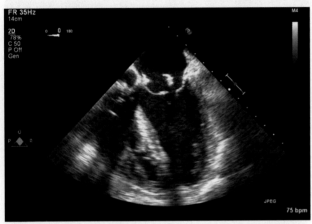

Figure 54-1.

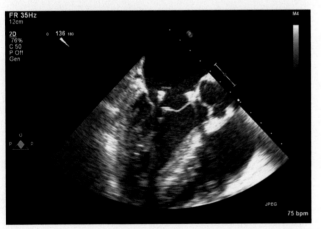

Figure 54-2.

QUESTION 1. What is the linear echo density in the left atrium in Figures 54-1 and 54-2 and Videos 54-1 and 54-2?

    A. A myxoma

    B. A calcific mitral annulus

    C. An artifact

    D. A mitral annuloplasty ring

Answers

ANSWER 1: *D.* There is no myxoma, no calcification of the annulus, and no artifact, but there is a dehisced annuloplasty ring as shown in Figure 54-3, which is a 3D transesophageal echocardiogram (TEE) image from the same patient. *Arrows* are indicating posterior mitral annulus. Mitral annuloplasty ring used for mitral valve repair is dehisced from this portion of the annulus.

3D TEE provides additional information compared with 2D TEE as seen in this case.

With 2D TEE, the entire structure of the mitral valvular annuloplasty ring relative to the mitral annulus could not be appreciated, and ring dehiscence was thus difficult to diagnose.

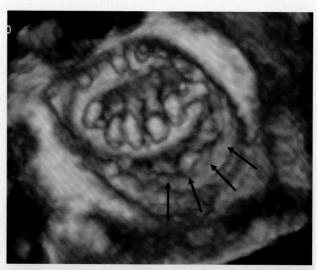

Figure 54-3.

Suggested Readings

Caiani EG, Fusini L, Veronesi F, et al. Quantification of mitral annulus dynamic morphology in patients with mitral valve prolapse undergoing repair and annuloplasty during a 6-month follow up. *Eur J Echocardiogr.* 2011;12:375–383.

Kronzon I, Sugeng L, Perk G, et al. Real-time 3-dimensional transesophageal echocardiography in the evaluation of post-operative mitral annuloplasty ring and prosthetic valve dehiscence. *J Am Coll Cardiol.* 2009;53:1543–1547.

CASE 55

Shortness of Breath and Palpitations

A 67-year-old man complains of shortness of breath and palpitations. He had robotic mitral valvular surgery 1 year ago.

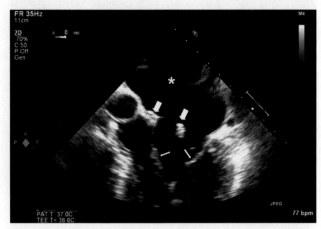

Figure 55-1.

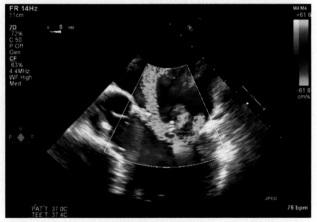

Figure 55-2.

QUESTION 1. Based on this 2D three-chamber transesophageal echocardiogram (TEE) view (Fig. 55-1), the patient has:

- A. A vegetation on the mitral valve
- B. A bioprosthetic mitral valve
- C. A mitral valve ring
- D. A mechanical mitral valve

QUESTION 2. See Figure 55-2. The mitral regurgitation (MR) is:

- A. Severe and central through the mitral valve (i.e., valvular)
- B. Severe and paravalvular
- C. Severe, both valvular and paravalvular
- D. Moderate, both valvular and paravalvular

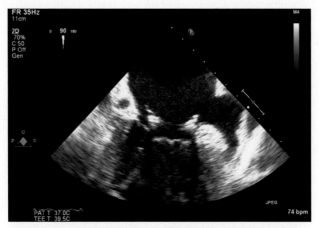

Figure 55-3.

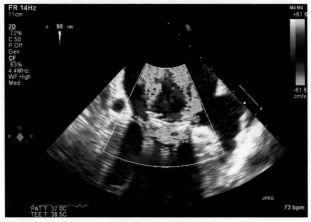

Figure 55-4.

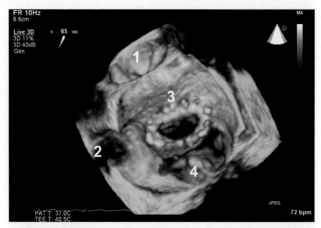

Figure 55-5.

QUESTION 3. See Figures 55-3 and 55-4. The paravalvular MR is located:

   A. Anteriorly

   B. Inferiorly

   C. Anteriorly and inferiorly

   D. Laterally

   E. Medially and laterally

QUESTION 4. This 3D TEE left atrial view (Fig. 55-5) shows:

   A. A dehisced mitral valve ring only attached posteriorly

   B. A dehisced mitral valve ring only attached anteriorly

   C. Posterior mitral leaflet prolapse

   D. Anterior mitral leaflet prolapse

   E. A dehisced mitral valve ring only attached anteriorly and posterior mitral leaflet prolapse

Answers

ANSWER 1: **C.** The patient has a mitral valve ring after mitral valve repair. The *asterisk* depicts an enlarged left atrium. The two *block arrows* point to the medial and the lateral portion of the mitral ring. Below the ring is the native mitral valve with *thin arrows* pointing to the anterior (*left*) and the posterior leaflet (*right*).

ANSWER 2: **C.** There is severe MR through both of the mitral leaflets as demonstrated by a medially directed jet toward the center of the picture. There also appears to be two jets of paravalvular MR on the lateral aspect of the valve. The lateral position of the ring is still seen as a bright echo density separating the valvular from the paravalvular jets.

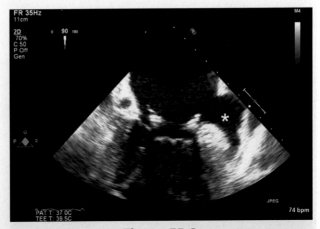

Figure 55-6.

ANSWER 3: **C.** These images (Figs. 55-6 and 55-7) are obtained in the two-chamber view (bicommissural view) at 90° and therefore showing the anterior aspect (to the right) and the inferior aspect (to the left) of the valve (*arrows*). The *asterisk* points to the left atrial appendage, an anterior structure that may assist one in determining the orientation of the image.

ANSWER 4: **E.** This 3D TEE surgical view depicts the aortic valve around 11 to 12 o'clock (*1*), and the left atrial appendage to the left at 9 o'clock (*2*). Central in the picture is the mitral valve ring, which is seen to be only attached anteriorly toward the aortic valve (*3*). Below the ring, a large P2 prolapsed segment is visualized (*4*).

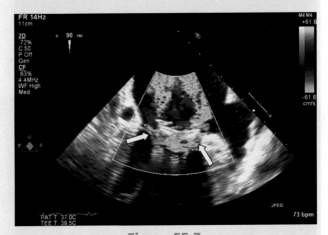

Figure 55-7.

Suggested Reading

Kronzon I, Sugeng L, Perk G, et al. Real-time 3-dimensional transesophageal echocardiography in the evaluation of post-operative mitral annuloplasty ring and prosthetic valve dehiscence. *J Am Coll Cardiol.* 2009;53:1543–1547.

Dyspnea, Orthopnea, and Pedal Edema

A 67-year-old man with a history of hypertension presents with 3 months of increasing dyspnea, orthopnea, and lower extremity edema. His transthoracic echocardiogram is shown in Figures 56-1 to 56-3.

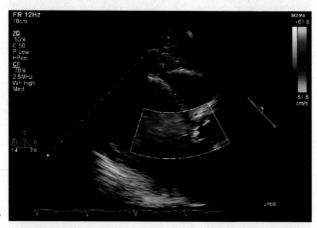

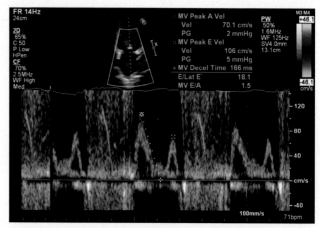

Figure 56-1A,B.

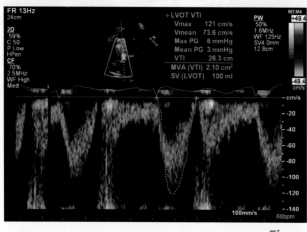

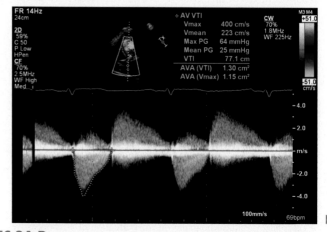

Figure 56-2A,B.

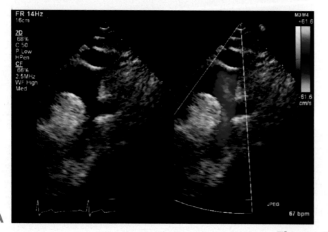

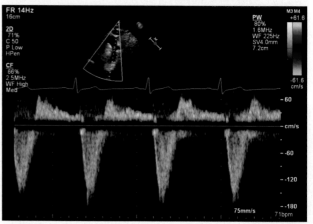

Figure 56-3A,B.

QUESTION 1. All of the following would support a diagnosis of severe aortic regurgitation (AR) *except*:

A. Jet width > 65% left ventricular outflow tract (LVOT)
B. Regurgitant fraction > 50%
C. Regurgitant volume > 50 mL per beat
D. Holodiastolic flow reversal
E. None of the options

QUESTION 2. Is it reasonable to replace an aortic valve in an asymptomatic patient with severe AR, normal ejection fraction, and left ventricular (LV) end-systolic diameter > 55 mm?

A. Yes
B. No

QUESTION 3. On the echocardiogram images (Figs. 56-1 to 56-3), which of the following are found?

A. Rapid filling of ventricle
B. Early peak atrioventricular velocity–time integral (VTI)
C. High LVOT VTI
D. Flow reversal in descending aorta
E. Rapid filling of ventricle and flow reversal in descending aorta

Answers

ANSWER 1: C. A regurgitant volume > equal to 60 mL per beat is highly suggestive of severe AR and not 50 mL per beat (Table 56-1).

ANSWER 2: A. According to the 2006 American College of Cardiology/American Heart Association guidelines for management of patients with valvular heart disease, indications for aortic valve replacement in AR are as follows:

- Severe, symptomatic (Class I recommendation)
- Severe, asymptomatic, and:
  - Left ventricular ejection fraction (LVEF) < 50% (I)
  - LV end-diastolic > 75 mm (Class IIa recommendation) (> 70 if progressive [Class IIb recommendation])
  - LV end-systolic > 55 mm (Class IIa recommendation) (> 50 if progressive [Class IIb recommendation])
- Asymptomatic undergoing open-heart (Class IIa recommendation for severe, Class IIb recommendation for moderate)

ANSWER 3: E. Figure 56-1 shows a high E wave with a relatively short deceleration time, indicating rapid filling of the left ventricle. Figure 56-3B shows a holodiastolic flow reversal in the descending aorta, signifying severe AR (marked by the *arrow* in Fig. 56-4).

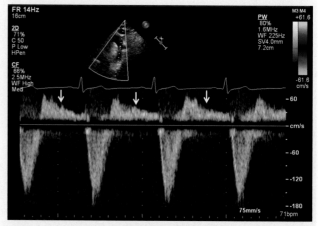

Figure 56-4.

TABLE 56-1. Qualitative and Quantitative Parameters Useful in Grading Aortic Regurgitation Severity

	Mild	Moderate		Severe
Structural parameters				
LA size	Normal	Normal or dilated		Usually dilated
Aortic leaflets	Normal or abnormal	Normal or abnormal		Abnormal/flail or wide coaptation defect
Doppler parameters				
Jet width in LVOT –Color Flow	Small in central jets	Intermediate		Large in central jets; variable in eccentric jets
Jet density –CW	Incomplete or faint	Dense		Dense
Jet deceleration rate – CW (PHT, ms)	slow > 500	Medium 500-200		Steep < 200
Diastolic flow reversal in descending aorta –PW	Brief, early diastolic reversal	Intermediate		Prominent holodiastolic reversal
Quantitative parameters				
VC width, cm	< 0.3	0.3–0.60		> 0.6
Jet width/LVOT width, %	< 25	25–45	46–64	≥ 65
Jet CSA/LVOT CSA, %	< 5	5–20	21–59	≥ 60
R Vol, ml/beat	< 30	30–44	45–59	≥ 60
RF, %	< 30	30–39	40–49	≥ 50
EROA, cm^2	< 0.10	0.10–0.19	0.20–0.29	≥ 0.30

Reprinted from Zoghbi WA, Enriquez-Sarano M, Foster E, et al. Recommendations for evaluation of the severity of native valvular regurgitation with two-dimensional and Doppler echocardiography. *J Am Soc Echocardiogr.* 2003;16:777–802, with permission from Elsevier.

Suggested Reading

Zoghbi WA, Enriquez-Sarano M, Foster E, et al. Recommendations for evaluation of the severity of native valvular regurgitation with two-dimensional and Doppler echocardiography. *J Am Soc Echocardiogr.* 2003;16:777–802.

CASE 57

Mitral Valve Reconstruction

A 68-year-old woman had mitral valve regurgitation due to a P2 prolapse. Her left ventricular ejection fraction was preserved, but she had pulmonary hypertension (pulmonary artery pressure > 65 mm Hg) and dyspnea (New York Heart Association [NYHA] class II to III). Therefore, she underwent surgery with a quadrangular resection of the P2 prolapse, and a mitral ring was implanted. After surgery, her symptoms did not remarkably improve. She still had dyspnea NYHA II-III. Six months after surgery, a transthoracic echocardiogram revealed severe mitral regurgitation, and a transesophageal echocardiogram (TEE) was done to define the etiology of the mitral regurgitation more precisely. The images (Videos 57-1 to 57-5 and Figs. 57-1 to 57-8) show the postsurgical echocardiogram findings.

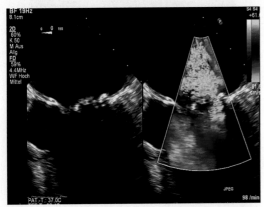

Figure 57-1. TEE four-chamber view without (*left*) and with color Doppler (*right*) in systole.

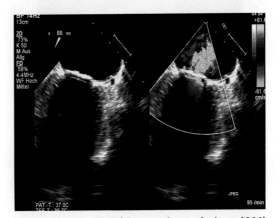

Figure 57-3. TEE bicommissural view (60°) in systole.

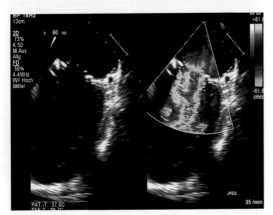

Figure 57-2. TEE bicommissural view (60°) in diastole.

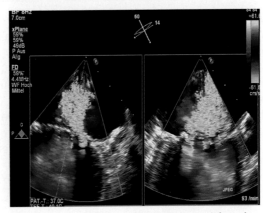

Figure 57-4. TEE x-plane views with color Doppler. Bicommissural view (*left*); long-axis view (*right*).

QUESTION 1. What causes the postsurgical mitral regurgitation (select all that apply)?

- A. Rupture of the mitral ring
- B. Lack of valve leaflet coaptation
- C. Paravalvular leak
- D. Rupture of the posterior leaflet
- E. A defect in the anterior leaflet

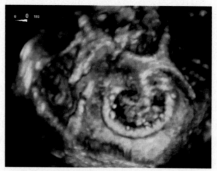

Figure 57-5. 3D TEE: Left atrial aspect of the mitral valve in systole.

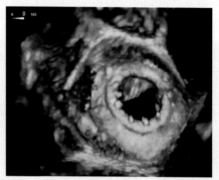

Figure 57-6. 3D TEE: Left atrial aspect of the mitral valve in diastole.

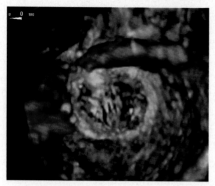

Figure 57-7. 3D TEE: Left ventricular aspect of the mitral valve in systole.

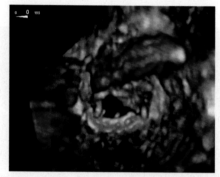

Figure 57-8. 3D TEE: Left ventricular aspect of the mitral valve in diastole.

Answers

ANSWER 1: B, E. The mitral regurgitation jets are clearly located within the borders of the surgically implanted ring; therefore, rupture of the mitral ring and paravalvular leak can be excluded as cause for the mitral regurgitation.

The implanted mitral ring covers the posterior leaflet completely, which is frequently the case. There is minimal posterior leaflet tissue, so rupture of the posterior leaflet can also be excluded. What can be observed is a lack of coaptation between the anterior and the posterior leaflet, best seen in the four-chamber view. In the intercommissural views, it can be seen that it is a very broad jet, indicating that the lack of coaptation is affecting the entire line of coaption. Therefore, lack of valve leaflet coaptation is correct.

In addition, the 3D images reveal a cleftlike lesion in the anterior leaflet, indicating a defect of this leaflet.

Due to these findings, the patient underwent reoperation and had a mitral valve replacement with a biological valve.

Suggested Reading

Kronzon I, Sugeng L, Perk G, et al. Real-time 3-dimensional transesophageal echocardiography in the evaluation of post-operative mitral annuloplasty ring and prosthetic valve dehiscence. *J Am Coll Cardiol.* 2009;53:1543–1547.

CASE 58

Mitral Valve Replacement with Anticoagulation Therapy

A 69-year-old woman has a history of mitral stenosis, chronic atrial fibrillation, and a past mitral valve commissurotomy in Russia.

She subsequently underwent mitral valve replacement and was treated with anticoagulation therapy.

The patient presented to the emergency room with dysuria and polyuria. She was discharged home the same day. Two days later, the patient came back to the emergency room because of slurred speech, which lasted for approximately 1 hour.

Upon physical examination, the patient was unarousable. Pulse was 110 beats per minute (irregularly irregular, atrial fibrillation) and blood pressure was 135/90 mm Hg. There was no jugular venous distention. There were normal heart sounds over precordium with a very clear prosthetic first sound audible. There was no diastolic murmur. Her lungs were clear to auscultation and percussion, and there was no peripheral edema noted.

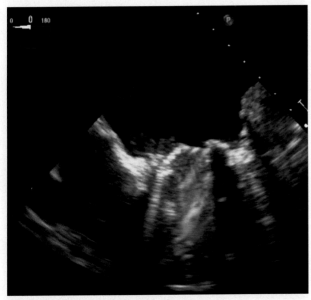

Figure 58-1.

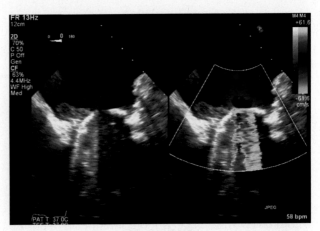

Figure 58-2.

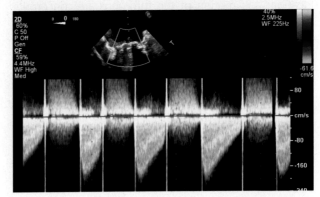

Figure 58-3. Continuous wave Doppler.

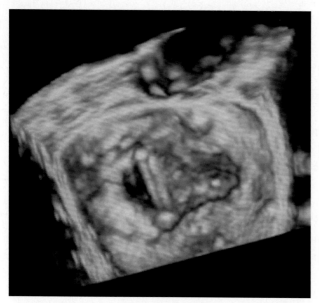

Figure 58-4.

QUESTION 1. Based on her transesophageal echocardiogram (TEE) shown in Figures 58-1 to 58-4 and Videos 58-1 to 58-3, what is the most likely cause of her slurred speech?

A. Hypertensive encephalopathy
B. Dementia
C. Diabetic ketoacidosis
D. Thromboembolism from a mechanical prosthetic mitral valve

Answers

ANSWER 1: D. There is a stenotic mechanical valve with a thrombosis and a nonmobile leaflet shown in the figures and videos. As such, thromboembolism is the most likely cause of the transient ischemic event of this patient as pointed out by the *arrow* in Figure 58-5.

Figure 58-4 and Video 58-3 are 3D TEE images that show an enface view of the mitral mechanical valve with a thrombus. This image is more informative than the 2D TEE (Figs. 58-1 and 58-2) as far as the shape, size, location, and motion of the thrombus are concerned. Also, the motion of the leaflets of the mechanical valve is clearly seen by 3D TEE imaging.

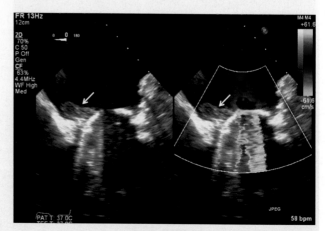

Figure 58-5.

Suggested Readings

Sugeng L, Shernan SK, Weinert L, et al. Real-time three-dimensional transesophageal echocardiography in valve disease: comparison with surgical findings and evaluation of prosthetic valves. *J Am Soc Echocardiogr.* 2008;21:1347–1354.

Tauras JM, Zhang Z, Taub CC. Incremental benefit of 3D transesophageal echocardiography: a case of a mass overlying a prosthetic mitral valve. *Echocardiography.* 2011;28:E106–E107.

CASE 59

Bulging of the Cardiac Silhouette

A 70-year-old man who had undergone a cardiac transplant 4 months previously suffered a loss of vision in the left eye, but he had no cardiac symptoms or abnormal findings upon physical examination. His chest x-ray showed a bulging of the cardiac silhouette to the right. An echocardiogram was ordered to further evaluate his cardiac status (Fig. 59-1 and Video 59-1).

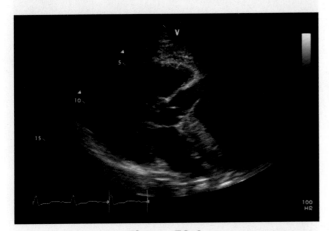

Figure 59-1.

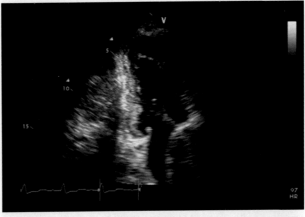

Figure 59-4.

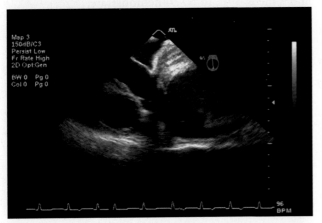

Figure 59-2.

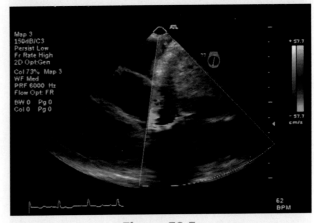

Figure 59-5.

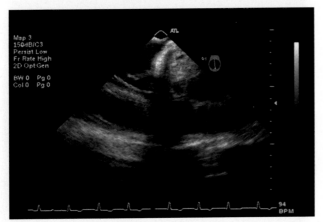

Figure 59-3.

QUESTION 1. This parasternal long-axis image (Fig. 59-1 and Video 59-1) shows:

A. A mass in the left atrium

B. A clot in the left atrium

C. Compression of the left atrium

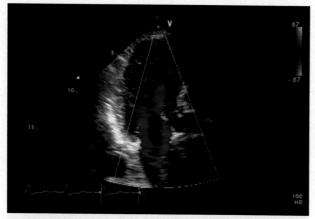

Figure 59-6.

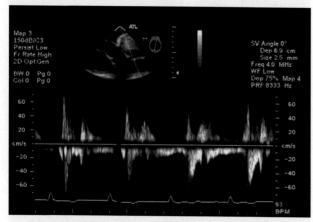

Figure 59-7.

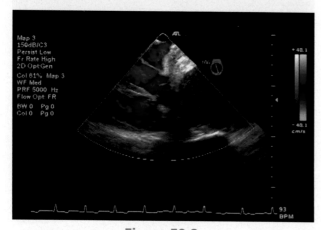

Figure 59-8.

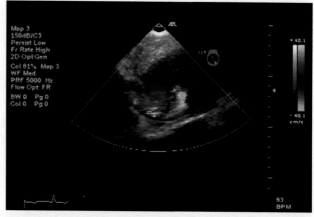

Figure 59-9.

QUESTION 2. What imaging test do you order next?

A. Transesophageal echocardiogram (TEE)
B. Magnetic resonance imaging (MRI)
C. Computed tomography (CT)
D. Any of the options

QUESTION 3. The TEE images (Figs. 59-2 to 59-9 and Videos 59-2 to 59-9) demonstrate:

A. An ascending aortic aneurysm
B. Communication between the mass and the ascending aorta, with a clot seen within the mass
C. An ascending aortic pseudoaneurysm
D. An extracardiac mass
E. Communication between the mass and the ascending aorta, with a clot seen within the mass and an ascending aortic pseudoaneurysm

Answers

ANSWER 1: C. The left atrium appears compressed from above.

ANSWER 2: D. As the compression of the atrium is superior, it needs an imaging modality that allows good assessment of the left atrium as well as the aorta. TEE, CT, and MRI are all sufficient for this purpose.

ANSWER 3: E. This is a pseudoaneurysm as there is clear disruption of the aortic wall.

The pseudoaneurysm contains a laminar clot and communicates with the aorta as seen in the transthoracic echocardiogram (Fig. 59-10A) and TEE (Fig. 59-10B) and on CT 3D reconstruction (Fig. 59-11).

This patient had a mycotic pseudoaneurysm due to *Aspergillus fumigatus.*

The most common cause of pseudoaneurysms is cardiac surgery, with the pseudoaneurysm originating at the suture line as it did in this case. Treatment is urgent surgical resection and repair.

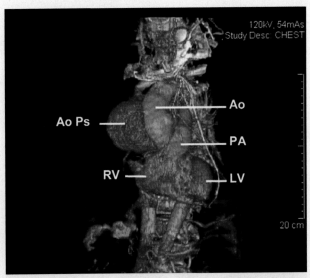

Figure 59-11. Contrast 3D CT angiogram of the aortic pseudoaneurysm. *Ao*, aorta; *Ao-Ps*, ascending aorta pseudoaneurysm; *LA*, left atrium; *LV*, left ventricle; *PA*, pulmonary artery; *RV*, right ventricle.

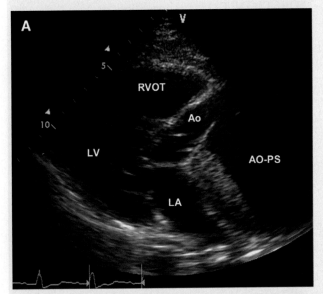
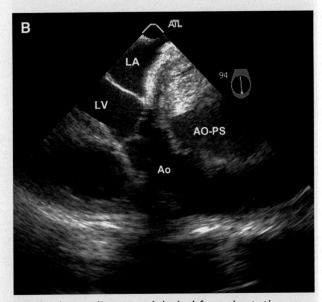

Figure 59-10. A. Transthoracic and **(B)** transesophageal echocardiograms labeled for orientation. *Ao*, aorta; *AO-PS*, ascending aorta pseudoaneurysm; *LA*, left atrium; *LV*, left ventricle; *RVOT*, right ventricular outflow tract.

Suggested Reading

Ronco F, Simsir S, Czer L, et al. Incidental finding by two-dimensional echocardiography of a mycotic pseudoaneurysm of the ascending aorta after orthotopic heart transplantation. *J Am Soc Echocardiogr.* 2010;23:580e1–e3.

Emergent Lysis of Adhesions

A 70-year-old woman is 1 day postoperative for emergent lysis of adhesions for small bowel obstruction. She develops pulmonary edema.

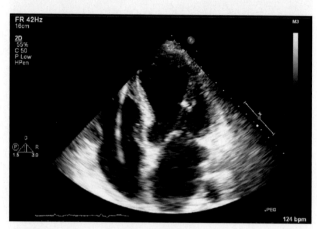

Figure 60-1.

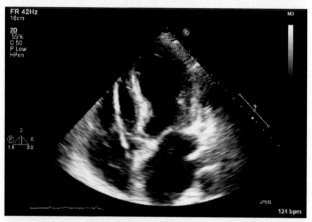

Figure 60-2.

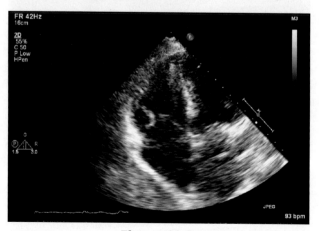

Figure 60-3.

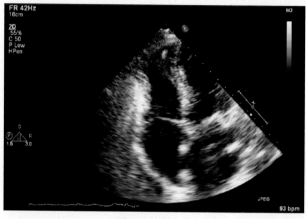

Figure 60-4.

QUESTION 1. Her echocardiogram (Figs. 60-1 to 60-6 and Videos 60-1 to 60-3) is consistent with:

   A Right coronary artery (RCA) infarction
   B. Left anterior descending (LAD) infarction
   C. RCA and LAD infarction
   D. Stress-induced cardiomyopathy

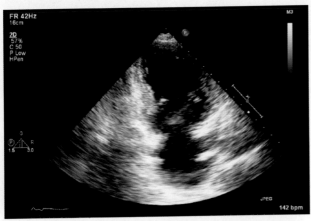

Figure 60-5.

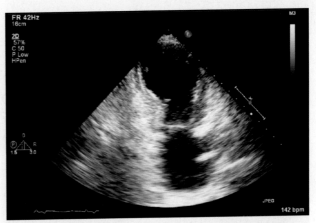

Figure 60-6.

Answers

ANSWER 1: D. Apical ballooning of both the left ventricle and right ventricle can be seen in these images. Thirty percent of stress-induced cardiomyopathy can be biventricular. Stress-induced cardiomyopathy occurs much more commonly in women.

Often referred to as Takotsubo cardiomyopathy, so named because the heart takes on the shape of a Japanese octopus trap due to ballooning of the ventricular apex, this form of cardiomyopathy is likely related to catecholamine surge and thus can be seen in a variety of situations including emotional upset, postsurgery, and septic shock.

Suggested Reading

Izumo M, Nalawadi S, Shiota M, et al. Mechanisms of acute mitral regurgitation in patients with Takotsubo cardiomyopathy: an echocardiographic study. *Circ Cardiovasc Imaging.* 2011;4:392–398.

Profound Hypertension after Hemodialysis

A 71-year-old woman with diabetes mellitus, hypertension, end-stage renal disease, status post mitral valve replacement, and history of bacteriemia presents with profound hypotension after hemodialysis.

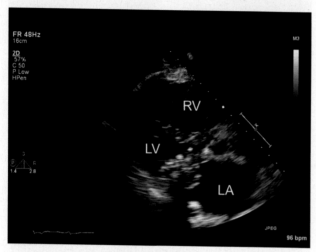

Figure 61-1.

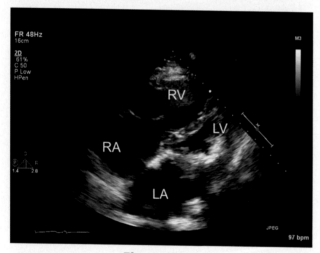

Figure 61-2.

QUESTION 1. Figures 61-1 and 61-2 (Videos 61-1 and 61-2) show:

A. A degenerated mechanical mitral valve prosthesis

B. A dilated right ventricle, along with a mass on the mitral valve

C. A dilated right ventricle, along with a tumor in the left atrium

D. A degenerated mechanical mitral valve prosthesis and a dilated right ventricle, along with a tumor in the left atrium

QUESTION 2. Figures 61-3 to 61-5 (Videos 61-3 and 61-4) demonstrate:

A. A mitral valve vegetation

B. Severe mitral regurgitation

C. Severe mitral stenosis

D. A mitral valve vegetation and severe mitral stenosis

E. A mitral valve vegetation and severe mitral regurgitation

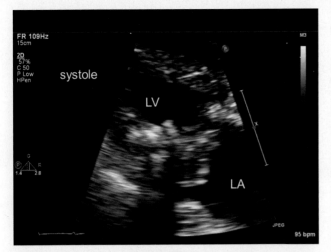

Figure 61-3.

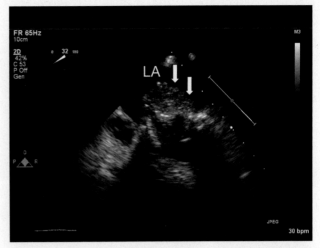

Figure 61-6.

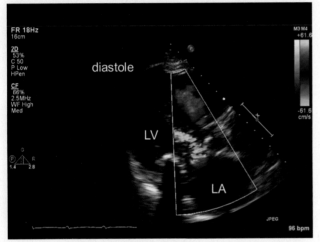

Figure 61-4.

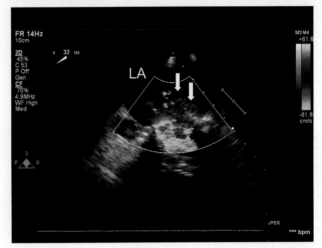

Figure 61-7.

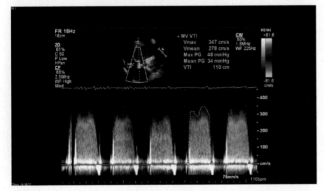

Figure 61-5.

QUESTION 3. The patient becomes somnolent. There are palpable pulses with a blood pressure of 40 mm Hg. Heart sounds are distant. There are no murmurs. What should you do next?

   A. Repeat the transthoracic echocardiogram—the gradient cannot be correct

   B. Perform a transesophageal echocardiogram (TEE) to better visualize the mass and to confirm that mitral stenosis is present

   C. Start intravenous (IV) antibiotics, IV pressors, and admit to the intensive care unit

   D. Emergent cardiac surgery for valve replacement

Answers

ANSWER 1: B. The images are obtained from the parasternal long-axis and subcostal views and demonstrate a markedly dilated right ventricle, a small left ventricle, and a large mass on the mitral valve. The mass partially obscures the valve structure, but there is no evidence of a mechanical mitral valve.

ANSWER 2: C. Figure 61-3 (Video 61-3) shows a large vegetation on a bioprosthetic mitral valve. Although the valve leaflets are not visible, the struts can be seen. Figure 61-4 (Video 61-4) shows a turbulent diastolic mitral inflow with large proximal isovelocity surface area in the left atrium, consistent with significant mitral stenosis. The continuous wave Doppler (Fig. 61-5) confirms critical mitral stenosis with a mean diastolic gradient of 34 mm Hg and a peak gradient of 48 mm Hg. There is no evidence of significant mitral regurgitation.

ANSWER 3: D. Emergent valve replacement is indicated. The patient is in cardiogenic shock due to mechanical obstruction of the mitral valve orifice most likely due to endocarditis. Although a TEE is indicated (Figs. 61-6 and 61-7 and Videos 61-5 and 61-6), this procedure should not delay the surgery and can be done intraoperatively.

Suggested Reading

Tiong IY, Novaro GM, Jefferson B, et al. Bacterial endocarditis and functional mitral stenosis: a report of two cases and brief literature review. *Chest.* 2002;122:2259–2262.

Mass Near Right Atrium

A 71-year-old man with a history of coronary artery bypass grafting (CABG) 20 and 10 years ago had a 2D and transesophageal echocardiogram (Figs 62-1 to 62-4).

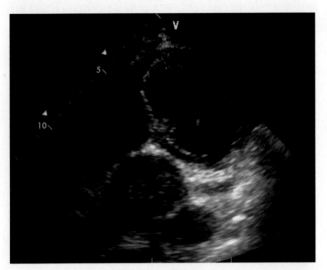

Figure 62-1.

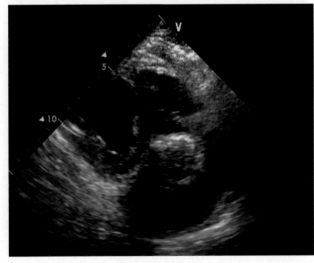

Figure 62-2.

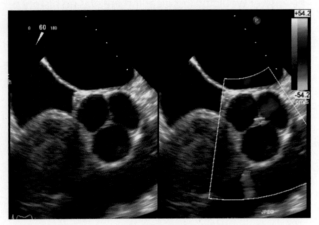

Figure 62-3.

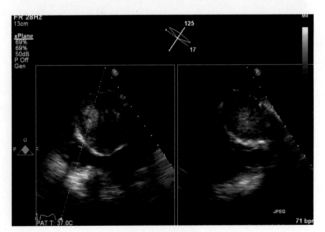

Figure 62-4.

QUESTION 1. What would be the next step?

A. Biopsy of the mass

B. Angiography

C. Nuclear stress test

D. Dobutamine stress echocardiogram

Answers

ANSWER 1: B. The mass appears to be circular and filled with clot making it likely to be a vein graft or right coronary artery aneurysm or pseudo-aneurysm. Thus, before performing a biopsy, angiography should be done first in this patient. A stress test is not indicated. The answer would be less clear if there was no history of CABG.

Angiography showed that the saphenous vein graft to the right coronary is patent and fills the posterior descending promptly. There was communication through this graft that has a slow filling of contrast throughout the cycle. The contrast fills through a septated area that gives the appearance of a thrombus that has been re-canalized. There is no apparent exit of the vascular mass, and there is no clear-cut neck that is noticed. The distal part of the graft before the anastomosis is lucent and looks somewhat as if it may be squashed by the mass that exists.

Suggested Reading

Jeon DS, Miyamoto T, Fontana G, et al. Pulmonary artery compression by a saphenous vein graft aneurysm and contrast echocardiography using an agitated mixture of ten percent air, ten percent blood, and ten percent saline. *J Am Soc Echocardiogr.* 2002;15:1529–1532.

CASE 63

Hypertrophic Cardiomyopathy with Lymphoma

A 71-year-old woman presents 2 years after successful alcohol septal ablation for hypertrophic cardiomyopathy. She was recently diagnosed with lymphoma and has subsequently developed new onset congestive heart failure (CHF).

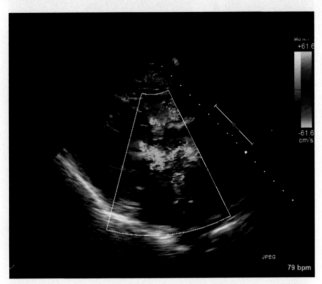

Figure 63-1. Transthoracic echocardiogram (TTE): Apical four-chamber view.

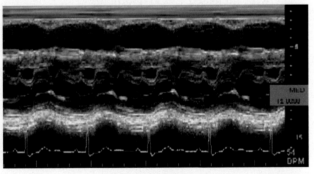

Figure 63-2.

QUESTION 1. Based on the parasternal long-axis and apical views (Fig. 63-1 and Video 63-1), which of the following is *most likely* correct?

  A. Patient has developed heart failure due to lymphoma infiltrating the myocardium
  B. CHF is associated with left ventricular dysfunction from chemotherapy
  C. Patient has had a recurrence of hypertrophic cardiomyopathy physiology with systolic anterior motion of the mitral valve (SAM), mitral regurgitation (MR), and left ventricular outflow tract (LVOT) gradient
  D. Heart failure due to a ventricular septal defect after alcohol septal ablation

QUESTION 2. Which of the following is not demonstrated on the motion (M)-mode echocardiogram (Fig. 63-2)?

  A. Asymmetric septal hypertrophy
  B. SAM
  C. Mitral annular calcification (MAC)
  D. Mitral stenosis

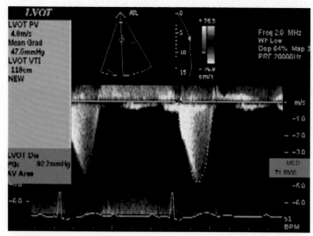

Figure 63-3. Five-chamber view. Continuous wave (CW) Doppler LVOT peak PGr = 92.2 mm Hg.

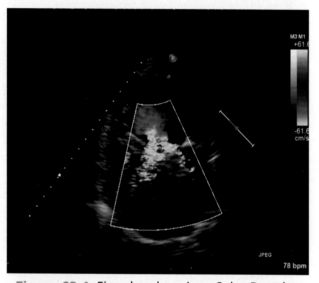

Figure 63-4. Five-chamber view. Color Doppler.

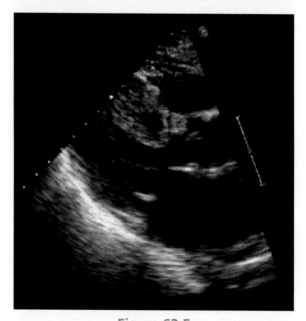

Figure 63-5.

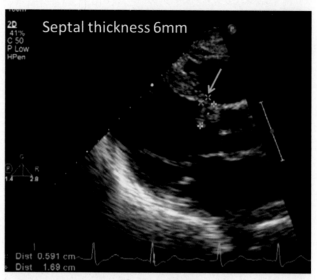

Figure 63-6.

QUESTION 3. See Figures 63-3 and 63-4. Which of the following is *not* true?

A. There is discrete membranous subaortic stenosis

B. There is dynamic LVOT gradient

C. There is severe eccentric MR

D. MR in hypertrophic cardiomyopathy (HCM) is generally posterolateral and often associated with increased LVOT gradients

QUESTION 4. Based on Figures 63-5 and 63-6, what is the treatment of choice for this patient?

A. Repeat alcohol septal ablation

B. Surgical myectomy

C. Mitral valve repair or replacement

D. Medical therapy with beta-blockers and disopyramide

Answers

ANSWER 1: C. Patient has had a recurrence of hypertrophic cardiomyopathy physiology with SAM, MR, and LVOT gradient.

ANSWER 2: D. Septum measures 2 cm, and the inferolateral wall measures 1 cm.

In Figure 63-7, the *yellow arrow* identifies SAM, and the *blue arrow* identifies MAC.

There is no evidence of mitral stenosis on the M-mode echocardiogram.

ANSWER 3: A. There is dynamic LVOT gradient. There is severe eccentric MR.

MR due to SAM in HCM is generally posterolateral and often associated with increased LVOT gradients.

There is no evidence of a discrete subaortic stenosis in this case.

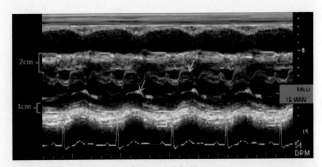

Figure 63-7.

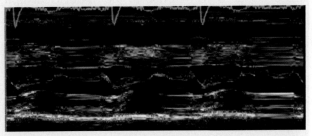

Figure 63-8.

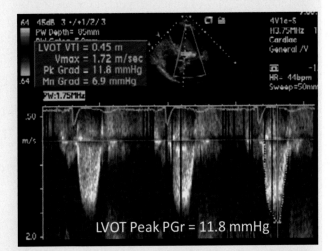

Figure 63-9. Rx disopyramide 400 mg, LVOT gradient ↓ from 92 to 12 mm Hg, MR from severe to mild, CHF resolved.

Answers

ANSWER 4: D. The treatment is medical therapy with beta-blockers and disopyramide. Figures 63-8 to 63-10 and Video 63-2 show the echocardiographic results after treatment with beta-blockers and disopyramide. This patient had reduction in MR and a significant decrease in the LVOT pressure gradient.

As the basal interventricular septum is only 6 mm on the 2D long-axis view, alcohol septal ablation and surgical myectomy are contraindicated. These procedures are generally contraindicated when the septal thickness is less or equal to 18 mm due to the risk of creating a ventricular septal defect with these interventions.

Mitral valve repair with an annuloplasty ring will not reduce the LVOT gradient. In a patient with advanced lymphoma and poor prognosis, surgery is relatively contraindicated.

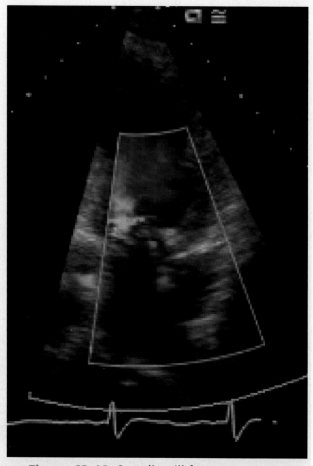

Figure 63-10. Systolic still frame–trace MR.

Suggested Reading

Fifer MA, Sigwart U. Controversies in cardiovascular medicine. Hypertrophic obstructive cardiomyopathy: alcohol septal ablation. *Eur Heart J.* 2011;32:1059–1064.

CASE 64

Moderate-to-Severe Mitral Regurgitation

A 71-year-old man complains of shortness of breath with chest pressure for 4 days. Past medical history includes end-stage renal disease on dialysis for the past 20 years, congestive heart failure, a biventricular pacemaker and implantable cardioverter-defibrillator, cirrhosis of the liver, and a history of ischemic cardiomyopathy with prior percutaneous coronary interventions.

Routine echocardiography demonstrates moderate-to-severe functional mitral regurgitation. Considering the risk of open heart surgery, a MitraClip (Abbott, Abbott Park, Illinois) procedure was performed to treat his mitral regurgitation.

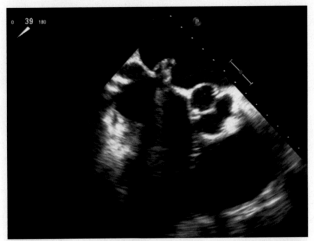

Figure 64-1.

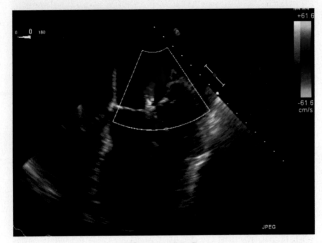

Figure 64-3.

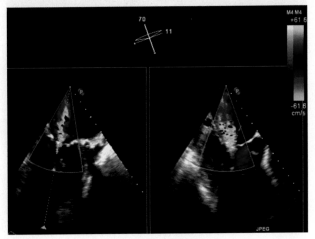

Figure 64-2.

QUESTION 1. As seen in Figures 64-1 to 64-3 and Videos 64-1 to 64-3, a MitraClip procedure was successfully performed with trivial residual mitral regurgitation.

Figure 64-4 and Video 64-4, a short-axis image in the level of the aortic valve with color Doppler, show:

  A. A ventricular septal defect
  B. Severe pulmonic valve regurgitation
  C. An atrial septal defect (ASD)
  D. Free wall perforation of the right atrium

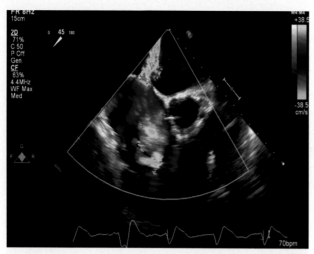

Figure 64-4.

QUESTION 2. After the procedure, the patient's O_2 saturation fell to 87% on 100% oxygen. What management should be considered in the catheterization laboratory?

A. Diuretics
B. Surgical closure of the ASD
C. 3D echocardiography
D. Percutaneous closure of the ASD

Answers

ANSWER 1: C. Due to the large catheter (22 F) used for the procedure, which crosses the atrial septum, a residual ASD was found after the procedure as shown in Figure 64-4 and Video 64-4.

ANSWER 2: D. Patients who develop significant right-to-left shunts and O_2 desaturation associated with catheterization laboratory transseptal procedures require acute closure of the shunt due to clinical deterioration, as these defects will not close spontaneously.

In this case, there was right-to-left shunting, the O_2 saturation fell to 87% on 100% oxygen, and the ASD was greater than 9 mm in diameter, warranting its closure, which was done percutaneously after the procedure.

The result was successful as seen in Figure 64-5 and Video 64-5.

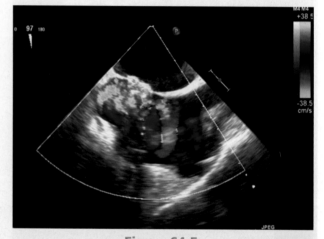

Figure 64-5.

Reference

Saitoh T, Izumo M, Furugen A, et al. Echocardiographic evaluation of iatrogenic atrial septal defect after catheter-based mitral valve clip insertion. *Am J Cardio.* 2012;109(12):1787–1791.

CASE 65

Mitral Valve Replacement

A 72-year-old woman from India underwent mitral valve replacement with a biological valve 2 years ago. Eight weeks later, she developed increasing dyspnea (New York Heart Association class II to III). A transesophageal echocardiogram (TEE) revealed recurrent mitral regurgitation and a paravalvular leak, which was suspected. The patient was referred for evaluation of transcatheter closure of a paravalvular mitral leak. A TEE study was performed (Videos 65-1 to 65-3 and Figs. 65-1 to 65-3).

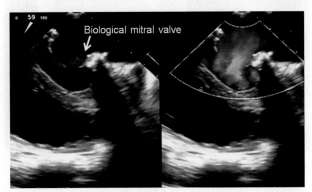

Figure 65-1. TEE: 59° in diastole.

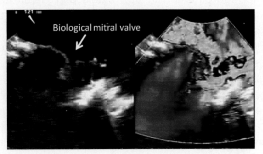

Figure 65-3. TEE: Long-axis (LAX) view, 120° in systole.

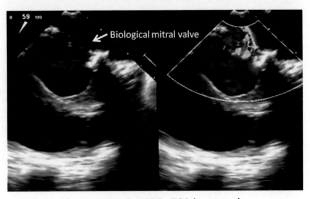

Figure 65-2. TEE: 59° in systole.

QUESTION 1. Which diagnosis is correct?

A. Mitral regurgitation due to a paravalvular leak in lateral location

B. Mitral regurgitation due to a paravalvular leak in medial location

C. Mitral regurgitation through the valve due to rupture of one leaflet at its base

D. Mitral regurgitation through the valve due to endocarditis and destruction of the valve

E. Mitral regurgitation through the valve due to early degeneration

Answers

ANSWER 1: C. The mitral regurgitation jet is clearly located within the surgically implanted mitral ring; therefore, a paravalvular leak can be excluded.

The morphology is seen best in the LAX view (120°). One regurgitation jet is very excentric and originates from the middle part, and another originates close to the inner mitral ring. A rupture of one leaflet at the base is present.

The regurgititation in the middle part is caused by the lack of coaptation due to the prolapsing ruptured leaflet.

The 3D TEE image (Fig. 65-4) shows the ruptured leaflet at the base in diastole; the edges of the leaflet are still connected to the ring.

Echocardiography provides detailed information about valve function and hemodynamics after mitral valve replacement, thus allowing early detection of structural valve deterioration.[1]

In this case, the bioprosthetic valve does not show any signs of degeneration. This suggests that this specific type of early structural valve deterioration, showing a leaflet rupture at the base of the leaflet, is likely due to a defective (rather than degenerated) bioprosthesis.

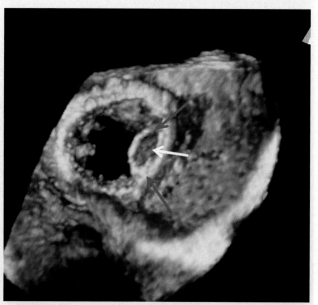

Figure 65-4. The *white arrow* marks the region where the leaflet is ruptured; the *red arrows* mark the edges where the leaflet is still connected to the ring.

Reference

1. Vesey JM, Otto CM. Complications of prosthetic heart valves. *Curr Cardiol Rep.* 2004;6:106–111.

CASE 66

Intestinal Bleeding and Atrioventricular Block

A 72-year-old woman was hospitalized due to intestinal bleeding. Her electrocardiogram showed a first-degree atrioventricular block. She had no dyspnea or chest pain and occasional palpitations. See Videos 66-1 and 66-2 and Figures 66-1 and 66-2.

An additional contrast study with agitated saline was performed. In Videos 66-3 and 66-4 and Figures 66-3 and 66-4, the contrast agent is applied once via a right cubital vein and once again via a left cubital vein.

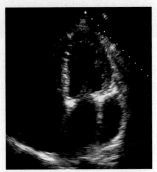

Figure 66-1. Transthoracic echocardiogram (TTE): Apical four-chamber view.

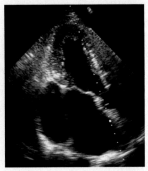

Figure 66-2. TTE: Apical three-chamber view.

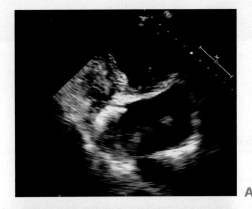

A

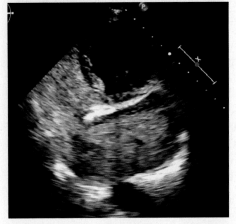

B

Figure 66-3A,B. TTE: Atypical apical four-chamber view. Agitated saline is injected into the right cubital vein. The agitated saline appears in the right atrium first, then the coronary sinus is opacificated.

QUESTION 1. What is the patient's diagnosis?

A. Coronary sinus aortic stenosis
B. Circumscribed pericardial effusion
C. Cor triatriatum sinister
D. Cor triatriatum dexter
E. Persistent left superior vena cava (PLSVC)

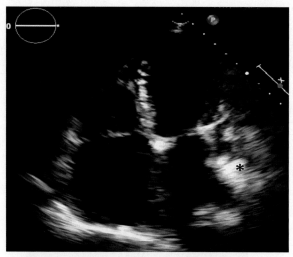
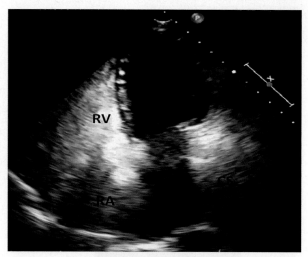

Figure 66-4. TTE: Apical four-chamber views. Agitated saline is applied via a left cubital vein. The coronary sinus (marked with a *black asterisk* on **A**) is opacificated first, then the right atrium and ventricle are opacificated (**B**). *RV*, right ventricle; *RA*, right atrium; *CS*, coronary sinus.

Answers

ANSWER 1: E. The patient has a PLSVC, which is considered the most common abnormality of the thoracic venous system.

The prevalence of PLSVC is approximately 0.3% of the general population.[1-3]

In isolation, as it appeared in our patient, this variation is considered benign. However, frequently, other congenital heart diseases (e.g., ventricular septal defect and atrioventricular septal defect)[4] are associated, which contribute to higher morbidity and mortality rates.

The left brachiocephalic vein does not develop fully, and the left upper limb, the head, and neck drain into the right atrium via the coronary sinus.

The diagnosis is confirmed by injecting agitated saline into the left arm vein, which leads to an opacification of the PLSVC and the dilated coronary sinus as the contrast study demonstrated in our patient.[5]

References

1. Pahwa R, Kumar A. Persistent left superior vena cava: an intensivist's experience and review of the literature. *South Med J.* 2003; 96(5):528–529.
2. Gonzalez-Juanatey C, Testa A, Vidan J, et al. Persistent left superior vena cava draining into the coronary sinus: report of 10 cases and literature review. *Clin Cardiol.* 2004;27(9):515–518.
3. Sarodia BD, Stoller JK. Persistent left superior vena cava: case report and literature review. *Respir Care.* 2000;45(4):411–416.
4. Biffi M, Boriani G, Fabretti L, et al. Left superior vena cava persistence in patients undergoing pacemaker or cardioverter defibrillator implantation. *Chest.* 2001;120:139–144.
5. Khouzam RN, Minderman D, D'Cruz IA. Review: echocardiography of the superior vena cava. *Clin Cardiol.* 2005;28:362–366.

Suggested Reading

Goyal SK, Punnam SR, Verma G, et al. Review: persistent left superior vena cava: a case report and review of literature. *Cardiovasc Ultrasound.* 2008;6:50.

CASE 67

Severe Mitral Regurgitation

A 72-year-old man with severe mitral regurgitation (MR) and a flail P3 scallop undergoes robotic mitral valve surgery. Transesophageal echocardiogram (TEE) images are obtained in the operating room after mitral valve surgery (Fig. 67-1 and Video 67-1).

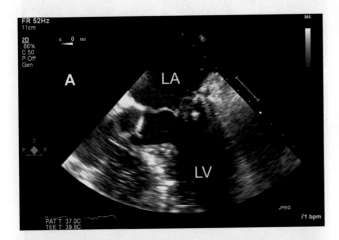

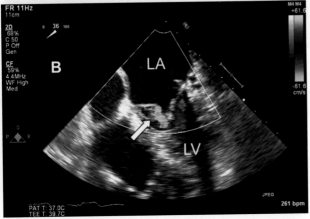

Figure 67-1. A. TEE five-chamber view: End-systole. **B.** TEE four-chamber view: Diastole.

QUESTION 1. What type of mitral valve surgery did the patient have?

   A. Mitral valve replacement with a bioprosthetic mitral valve

   B. Mitral valve repair

   C. Mitral valve replacement with a mechanical mitral valve

   D. Alfieri stitch

QUESTION 2. The color Doppler in Figure 67-1B (*arrow*) is due to:

   A. Residual MR

   B. Mitral stenosis after the repair

   C. Aortic regurgitation

   D. Systolic anterior motion (SAM) of the mitral apparatus with left ventricular outflow tract gradient

QUESTION 3. The following applies to the aortic regurgitation seen in Figure 67-2 and Video 67-2:

   A. The jet is eccentric, originating from the area between the right and the noncoronary cusps

   B. There appears to be a tear of the right coronary cusp

   C. The jet is eccentric and caused by a bicuspid aortic valve

   D. The jet is eccentric, originating from the area between the right and the noncoronary cusps, and there appears to be a tear of the right coronary cusp

   E. The jet is eccentric, originating from the area between the right and the noncoronary cusps, and the jet is eccentric caused by a bicuspid aortic valve

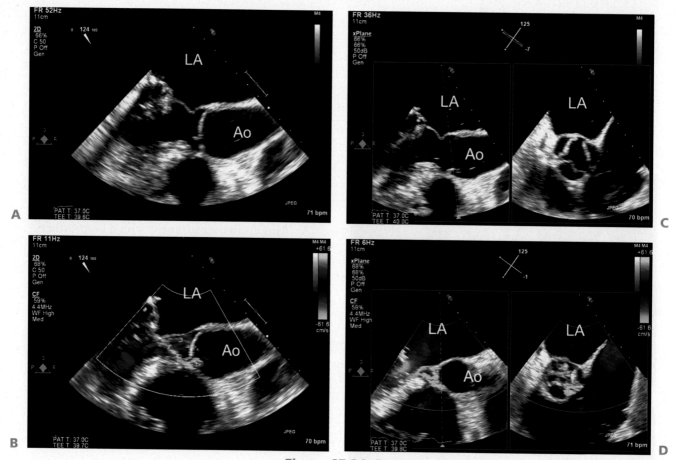

Figure 67-2A–D.

Answers

ANSWER 1: B. The valve was repaired using a partial annuloplasty ring and triangular resection of a flail P3 segment with closure of the posterior commissure and reattachment of the chords. The valve is still visibly myxomatous. There is no evidence of a bioprosthetic or mechanical valve. The Alfieri stitch would not be used for a P3 prolapse/flail segment.

ANSWER 2: C. It is always important to evaluate for residual MR and for the presence of mitral stenosis after repair. The color jet is seen in diastole on the ventricular side of the mitral valve and can therefore not be due to MR. Similarly, SAM is a systolic event and therefore also excluded. The absence of flow convergence on the atrial side excludes a jet due to mitral stenosis. The color flow represents the presence of new aortic regurgitation. Further imaging is required to better characterize the lesion and severity.

ANSWER 3: D. The images demonstrate a tricuspid aortic valve with a normal size aorta and a significant eccentric aortic regurgitation jet. In the short-axis view (Fig. 67-2D), the jet is seen originating from the area between the right and the noncoronary cusps and possibly involving a tear of the right cusp as seen by the origin of the color flow as well as by a filamentous structure (tear) in the long-axis view in Figure 67-2A. Figure 67-3 shows the location of the aortic cusps. The patient was placed back on pump, and the tear was successfully repaired.

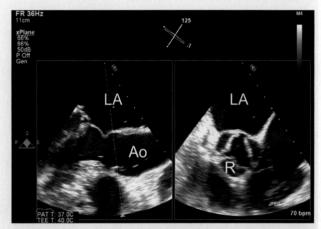

Figure 67-3. *Ao*, aorta; *LA*, left atrium; *R*, right coronary cusp.

Suggested Reading

O'Gara P, Sugeng L, Lang R. The role of imaging in chronic degenerative mitral regurgitation. *JACC Cardiovasc Imaging*. 2008;1:221–237

CASE 68

Symptomatic Aortic Stenosis

A 72-year-old man underwent aortic valve replacement 2 months ago for symptomatic severe aortic stenosis. He now presents with a 2-week history of fever, chills, rigors, and worsening fatigue. On physical exam, his blood pressure is 110/75 mm Hg, and pulse is 105 beats per minute and regular. Neck veins are flat, carotid pulses are normal, and lungs are clear to auscultation. Cardiac exam reveals a well-healed midline scar, a normal S1 and S2 with no S3 or S4 gallops. There is a 2/6 systolic ejection murmur in the left upper sternal border that radiates to the carotids. Extremities are warm with no peripheral edema.

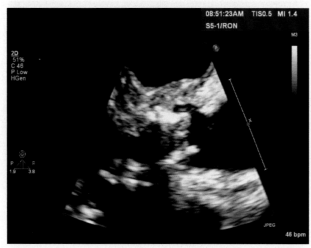

Figure 68-1. Transthoracic echocardiogram (TTE): Parasternal long-axis zoom.

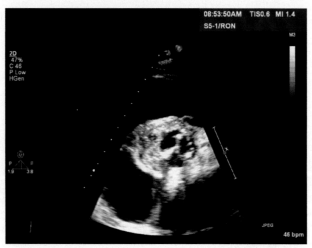

Figure 68-2. 3D TTE: Parasternal short axis.

QUESTION 1. Based on Figures 68-1 and 68-2 and Videos 68-1 to 68-4, the diagnosis is:

A. Mitral ring abscess
B. Aortic root abscess
C. Aortic valve dehiscence
D. Gerbode defect
E. All of the options

QUESTION 2. The most likely associated abnormal finding on his electrocardiogram is:

A. Left bundle branch block
B. Low QRS voltage
C. High QRS voltage
D. Atrioventricular (AV) block

QUESTION 3. After obtaining three sets of blood cultures, the best management strategy would be:

A. Intravenous (IV) ampicillin and gentamicin
B. IV vancomycin, gentamicin, and rifampin
C. Urgent aortic valve replacement
D. Transesophageal echocardiography
E. IV vancomycin, gentamicin, and rifampin; transesophageal echocardiography; and then urgent aortic valve replacement

Answers

ANSWER 1: B. The echocardiogram demonstrates a bioprosthetic valve in the aortic position. There is evidence of abnormal thickening around the aortic ring in the parasternal long-axis and short-axis views (Figs. 68-2 and 68-3 and Videos 68-3 and 68-4, marked with *arrows*). These findings, coupled with the clinical history, suggest the presence of an aortic ring abscess. Some degree of thickening around a bioprosthetic valve may represent normal postoperative change, so it is helpful to obtain a baseline TTE after aortic valve replacement to serve as a baseline for serial comparison.

ANSWER 2: D. The aortic ring is in close proximity to the AV node. Patients with aortic ring abscesses commonly develop AV block. The development of AV block is an ominous sign and implies rapid progression of the infection. Patients with suspected aortic valve endocarditis should have serial electrocardiography with close monitoring of the heart rate and conduction abnormalities such as prolongation of the PR interval and/or QRS duration as well as heart block.

ANSWER 3: E. After starting empiric antibiotic therapy for prosthetic valve endocarditis, the patient should undergo transesophageal echocardiography and urgent aortic valve replacement with debridement of the aortic ring abscess. The currently recommended empiric regimen for prosthetic valve endocarditis is vancomycin, gentamicin, and rifampin. Aortic ring abscesses responds poorly to antibiotics alone. Prompt surgical intervention is warranted and often lifesaving.

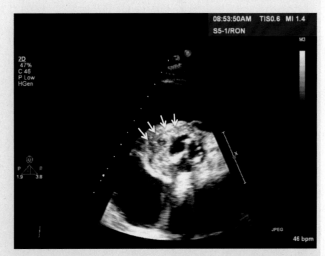

Figure 68-3.

Suggested Reading

David TE, Komeda M, Brofman PR. Surgical treatment of aortic root abscess. *Circulation.* 1989;80:1269–1274.

Paroxysmal Nocturnal Dyspnea and Worsening Pedal Edema

A 73-year-old man presents with a 6 months history of worsening exertional fatigue and dyspnea on exertion. More recently, he has developed paroxysmal nocturnal dyspnea and worsening pedal edema. Upon physical examination, there is jugular venous distension to the angle of the jaw. Lungs are clear to auscultation. Cardiac exam reveals a diffuse point of maximum impulse in the fifth intercostal space. S1 is normal, and there is an increase in the P2 component of S2. There is a loud third heart sound and a 2/6 holosystolic murmur in the apex radiating to the axilla. Extremities reveal 3+ pedal edema.

An electrocardiogram (Fig. 69-1) and 2D echocardiogram (Figs. 69-2 to 69-6 and Videos 69-1 to 69-3) are performed.

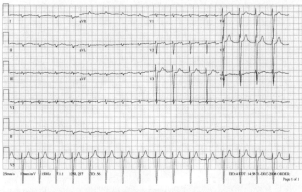

Figure 69-1.

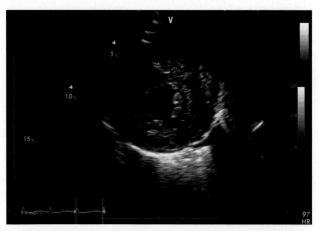

Figure 69-3. TTE: Parasternal short-axis view.

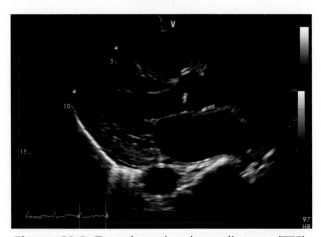

Figure 69-2. Transthoracic echocardiogram (TTE): Parasternal long-axis view.

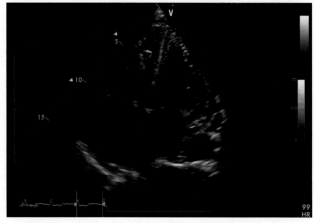

Figure 69-4. TTE: Apical four-chamber view.

QUESTION 1. What is the most appropriate next step to confirm the diagnosis?

A. Right and left heart catheterization
B. Myocardial contrast echocardiography
C. Serum protein electrophoresis
D. Urine protein electrophoresis
E. Abdominal fat pad biopsy

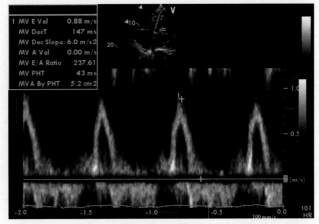

Figure 69-5.

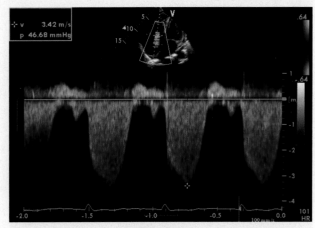

Figure 69-6.

Answers

ANSWER 1: E. This patient has findings suggestive of cardiac amyloidosis with a restrictive cardiomyopathy. Amyloidosis can be caused by an underlying paraprotein-emia such as multiple myeloma (light-chain amyloidosis) or a chronic inflammatory condition (AA amyloidosis [amyloidosis related to inflammatory diseases]).

The least invasive initial test to confirm the diagno-sis of systemic amyloid is an abdominal fat pad biopsy. The appearance of apple-green birefringence on Congo red staining is a characteristic of amyloidosis. However, it has a limited sensitivity, and some patients will require myocardial biopsy to confirm the diagnosis.

Suggested Reading

Falk RH. Diagnosis and management of the cardiac amyloidoses. *Circulation.* 2005;112:2047–2060.

CASE 70

End-stage Renal Disease and Hypertension

A 73-year-old man with end-stage renal disease due to long-standing hypertension has a routine echocardiogram performed, and the images in Figures 70-1 and 70-2 are recorded.

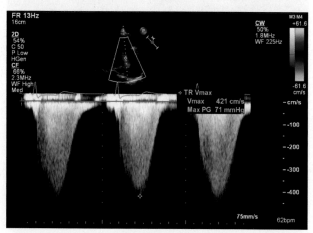

Figure 70-1.

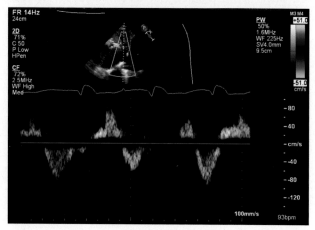

Figure 70-2.

QUESTION 1. What is the valvular lesion and its severity?

- A. Mitral regurgitation, moderate
- B. Mitral regurgitation, severe
- C. Tricuspid regurgitation, moderate
- D. Tricuspid regurgitation, severe

QUESTION 2. All of the following are correct regarding various measures of tricuspid regurgitation (TR) severity *except*:

- A. Right ventricular (RV)/right atrial (RA)/inferior vena cava size: May be normal in acute TR
- B. Jet area: Overestimates severity in eccentric jets
- C. Jet density: Depends on RA pressure and RV relaxation, tricuspid valve area, and atrial fibrillation
- D. Hepatic vein flow: Systolic flow reversal is sensitive for severe TR

QUESTION 3. Which is more sensitive for severe TR?

- A. Jet width
- B. Hepatic vein flow reversal

QUESTION 4. An accepted cutoff for the RA-RV pressure gradient that requires further evaluation for pulmonary hypertension is:

- A. 30 mm Hg
- B. 40 mm Hg
- C. 50 mm Hg
- D. 60 mm Hg

Answers

ANSWER 1: D. The Doppler shows a TR jet that is both holosystolic and quite dense. There is systolic flow reversal in the hepatic vein. These are consistent with severe TR.

ANSWER 2: B. Jet area underestimates TR in eccentric jets.

ANSWER 3: A. Jet width > 0.7 cm has a sensitivity of 89% and specificity of 93%. However, it can underestimate TR in 20% to 30%.

Systolic flow reversal is sensitive (80%) for severe TR and likely also very specific. However, it is influenced by RA pressure, atrial fibrillation, RV relaxation, and the phase of the respiratory cycle.

ANSWER 4: B. In the absence of other potential etiologies of pulmonary hypertension (PH), such as left heart disease or advanced lung disease, an estimated RV systolic pressure of greater than 40 mm Hg generally warrants further evaluation in the patient with unexplained dyspnea.

Suggested Readings

McLaughlin W, Archer SL, Badesch DB, et al. ACCF/AHA 2009 expert consensus document on pulmonary hypertension: a report of the American College of Cardiology foundation task force on expert consensus documents and the American Heart Association developed in collaboration with the American College of Chest Physicians; American Thoracic Society, Inc.; and the Pulmonary Hypertension Association. *J Am Coll Cardiol.* 2009;53: 1573–1619.

Zoghbi WA, Enriquez-Sarano M, Foster E, et al. American Society of Echocardiography: recommendations for evaluation of the severity of native valvular regurgitation with two-dimensional and Doppler echocardiography: a report from the American Society of Echocardiography's Nomenclature and Standards Committee and The Task Force on Valvular Regurgitation, developed in conjunction with the American College of Cardiology Echocardiography Committee, the Cardiac Imaging Committee, Council on Clinical Cardiology, the American Heart Association, and the European Society of Cardiology Working Group on Echocardiography. *Eur J Echocardiogr.* 2003;4(4):237–261.

CASE 71

Aortic Stenosis and Atrial Fibrillation

A 74-year-old woman with severe aortic stenosis and atrial fibrillation (AFIB) is referred for aortic valve replacement. See Figures 71-1 to 71-3 and Videos 71-1 to 71-3.

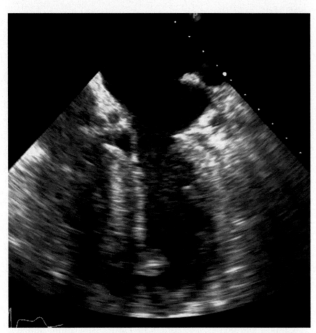

Figure 71-1.

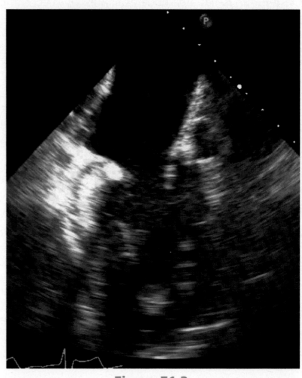

Figure 71-3.

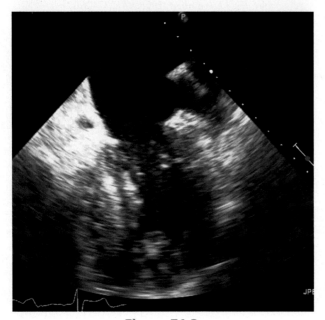

Figure 71-2.

QUESTION 1. In addition to aortic stenosis, the patient also has:

   A. Left atrial appendage thrombus
   B. Apical thrombus
   C. Endocarditis
   D. Left ventricular (LV) myxoma
   E. LV papillary fibroelastoma (PFE)

Answers

ANSWER 1: E. This is a very unusual case of LV PFE. Primary cardiac tumors are very rare, and the most common is myxoma, which would make this the most likely diagnosis of this incidental finding in our patient. PFE is the third most common primary tumor of the heart but is most frequently seen on the aortic or mitral valve. PFE may embolize and cause distant embolization or myocardial infarctions due to embolization to the coronary arteries. Although the patient has AFIB, there is no evidence of a thrombus in the left atrial appendage. LV thrombus is very unlikely, given the normal LV size and function without evidence of segmental wall motion abnormalities. Although metastatic disease is more common than primary cancers of the heart, the patient is in overall good health without evidence of cancer in other places. The LV mass is seen in multiple views and does not represent an artifact (Figs. 71-4 to 71-8 and Videos 71-4 and 71-5).

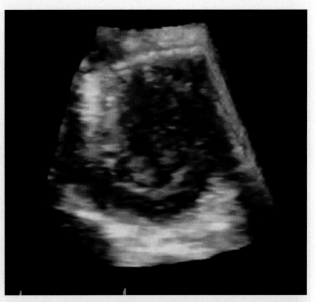

Figure 71-5.

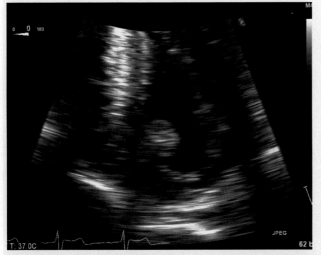

Figure 71-4.

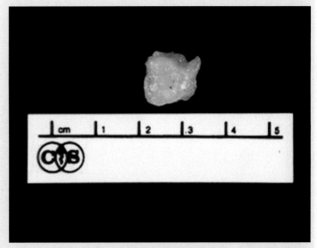

Figure 71-6.

Answers

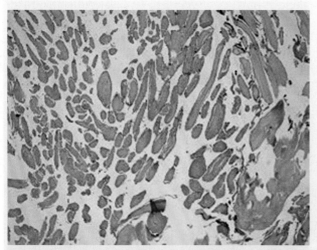

Figure 71-7.

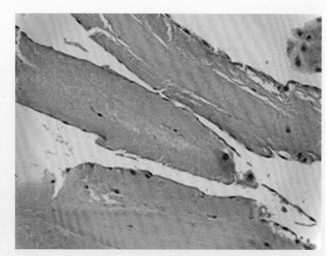

Figure 71-8.

Suggested Reading

Sydow K, Schrepfer S, Franzen O, et al. Coincidence of aortic valve stenosis and regurgitation and multiple cardiac papillary fibroelastomas in a young male adult. *J Thorac Cardiovasc Surg.* 2007;133:564–565.

Heart Murmur, Systemic Hypertension, and History of Cerebrovascular Accident

A 75-year-old man with a heart murmur since childhood, hypertension, and a history of a cerebrovascular accident had an echocardiogram to evaluate his heart murmur.

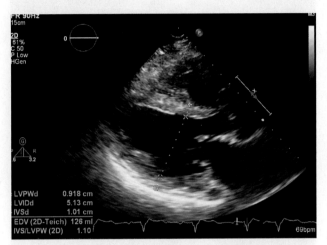

Figure 72-1.

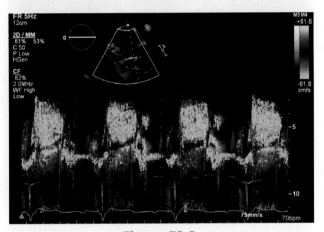

Figure 72-2.

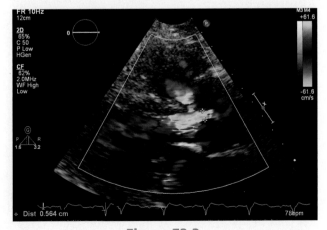

Figure 72-3.

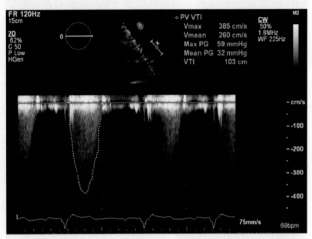

Figure 72-4. Continuous wave Doppler across right ventricular outflow tract (RVOT).

QUESTION 1. The 2D echocardiogram (Fig. 72-1) and the color motion (M)-mode echo (Fig. 72-2) show (select all that apply):

A. Severe tricuspid regurgitation
B. A ventricular septal defect (VSD)
C. An overriding aorta
D. Eisenmenger syndrome

QUESTION 2. Figure 72-3 demonstrates:

A. A double outlet right ventricle (RV)
B. An atrial septal defect
C. Aortic regurgitation
D. Truncus arteriosus

QUESTION 3. Figures 72-1 to 72-4 are consistent with which of the following in this 75-year-old man?

A. Nonrestricted VSD
B. Gerbode defect
C. Truncus arteriosus
D. Endocardial cushion defect
E. Tetralogy of Fallot

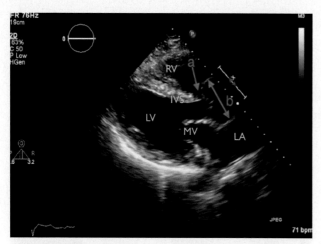

Figure 72-5. Parasternal long-axis view demonstrating: **(A)** the VSD and **(B)** overriding aorta. *IVS*, intraventricular septum; *LA*, left atrium; *LV*, left ventricle; *MV*, mitral valve; *RV*, right ventricle.

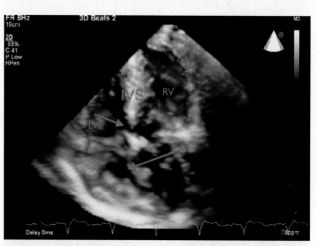

Figure 72-7. 3D TTE of the apical three-chamber view demonstrating the VSD (*single arrow*) and the overriding aorta (*double arrow*). *iVS*, intraventricular septum; *LA*, left atrium; *LV*, left ventricle; *RV*, right ventricle.

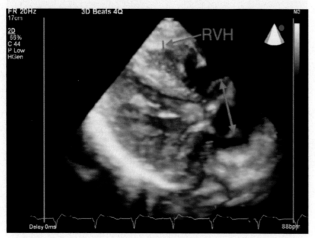

Figure 72-6. 3D transthoracic echocardiogram (TTE) from the parasternal long-axis view demonstrating normal size left ventricular cavity, right ventricular hypertrophy (*RVH*), and overriding aorta (*double arrows*).

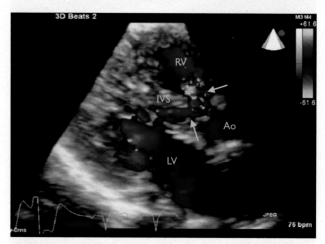

Figure 72-8. 3D TTE parasternal long-axis view with color Doppler demonstrating bidirectional flow (*yellow arrows*) across the VSD. *Ao*, aorta; *IVS*, interventricular septum; *LV*, left ventricle; *RV*, right ventricle.

QUESTION 4. Which of the following factors are thought to be associated with improved longevity and minimal symptoms in uncorrected (unoperated) tetralogy of Fallot (see Figs. 72-5 to 72-10)?

A. A hypoplastic pulmonary artery with slow development of subpulmonary obstruction[1]

B. Left ventricular hypertrophy (LVH)

C. Extracardiac shunts

D. All of the options

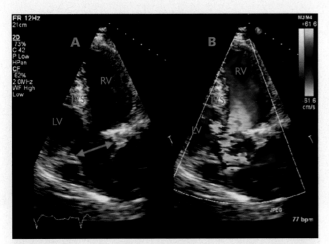

Figure 72-9. Apical five-chamber view (**A**) demonstrating the overriding aorta (*double arrows*) and color Doppler (**B**) demonstrating bidirectional flow across the VSD. *IVS*, interventricular septum; *LV*, left ventricle; *RV*, right ventricle.

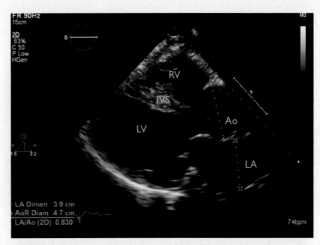

Figure 72-10. Parasternal long-axis view demonstrating the overriding aorta (*Ao*). *IVS*, interventricular septum; *LA*, left atrium; *LV*, left ventricle; *RV*, right ventricle.

Answers

ANSWER 1: B, C. An overriding aorta is seen in Figure 72-1. The color M-mode (Fig. 72-2) demonstrates flow through the VSD (see also Fig. 72-11).

ANSWER 2: C. This diastolic frame demonstrates aortic regurgitation.

ASNWER 3: E. There is an overriding aorta, a VSD, an RVOT obstruction, as well as RVH (see Figs. 72-5 to 72-10 and 72-12 and Videos 72-1 and 72-2).

ANSWER 4: D. There are three factors that are associated with improved longevity in tetralogy of Fallot:

1) A hypoplastic pulmonary artery with slow development of subpulmonary obstruction[1]
2) LVH that is thought to act by delaying of shunting from the right-to-left ventricle.[2,3] LVH may be a late development in the natural history of Fallot, and any beneficial effect may not be seen until adult life. Such balanced hemodynamics as in this case are unusual.
3) Extracardiac shunts including patent ductus arteriosus[4]—reported in the oldest survivor who died at age 77[5]—or systemic to pulmonary artery shunting via internal mammaries[6]

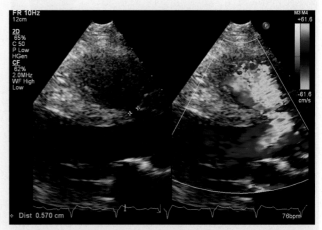

Figure 72-11.

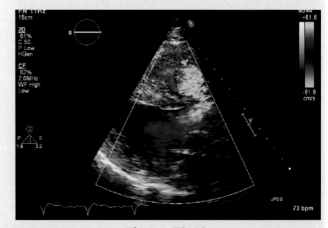

Figure 72-12.

References

1. Meindok H. Longevity in the tetralogy of Fallot. *Thorax.* 1964; 19:12–15.
2. Bowie EA. Longevity in tetralogy and tetralogy of Fallot. Discussion of cases in patients surviving 40 years and presentation of two further cases. *Am Heart J.* 1961;62:125–32.
3. Chin J, Bashour T, Kabbani S. Tetralogy of Fallot in the elderly. *Clin Cardiol.* 1984;7:453–456.
4. Nottestad SY, Slife DM, Rubal BJ, et al. Tetralogy of Fallot in a 71-year-old patient with new onset hypoxemia. *Cathet Cardiovasc Diagn.* 1993;28:335–338.
5. Thomas SHL, Bass P, Pambakian H, et al. Cyanotic tetralogy of Fallot in a 77-year-old man. *Postgrad Med J.* 1987;63:361–362.
6. Liberthson RR, Miller SW, Drew F, et al. Congenital extracardiac shunts with tetralogy of Fallot. *Cardiovasc Intervent Radiol.* 1981;4:131–135.

Recurrent Episodes of Bronchitis and Pneumonia

*A*79-year-old woman has a history of shortness of breath, bronchial asthma, and bronchiectasis associated with recurrent episodes of bronchitis and pneumonia.

She developed left upper anterior pleuritic chest pain. Her blood pressure was 143/75 mm Hg, pulse was 105 beats per minute, respiration was 18 breaths per minute, and O_2 saturation is 98% on room air. Her chest x-ray showed new small bilateral pleural effusions. White blood cell count was 7100 cells/ml, hemoglobin was 11.5 gr/dl, natriuretic peptide assay was 637 pg/ml, and troponin was 0.43 µg/L. The electrocardiogram (ECG) demonstrated inverted T waves over the anterior precordium (Fig. 73-1).

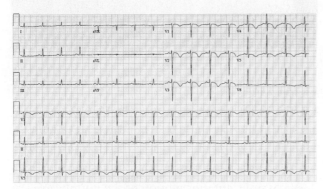

Figure 73-1.

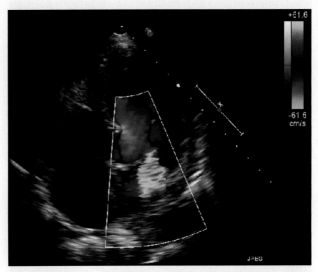

Figure 73-3.

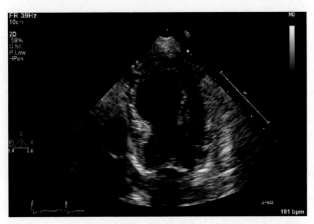

Figure 73-2.

QUESTION 1. The echocardiograms (Figs. 73-2 and 73-3) show:

- A. Apical akinesis or dyskinesis with significant mitral regurgitation (MR)
- B. Apical hypokinesis without significant MR
- C. Diffuse hypokinesis
- D. Normal left ventricular (LV) size and function

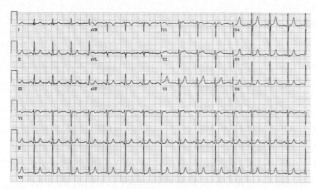

Figure 73-4.

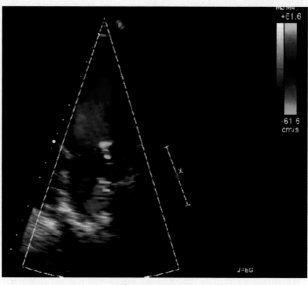

Figure 73-6.

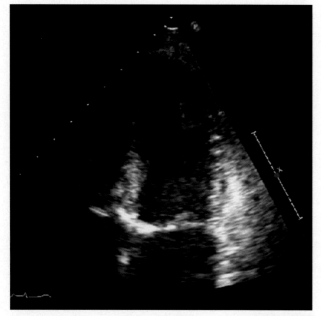

Figure 73-5.

QUESTION 2. After 3 weeks, the ECG normalized and LV function and MR improved as shown in Figures 73-4 to 73-6. Cardiac catheterization showed normal coronary arteries. What is the cause of MR?

A. Systolic anterior motion of the mitral valve (SAM)
B. Congenital
C. Endocarditis
D. Tethering of the mitral apparatus

Answers

ANSWER 1: A. Significant MR and apical akinesis or dyskinesis are noted.

ANSWER 2: D. Tethering is noted in Figure 73-2, which subsequently improved as shown in Figure 73-5 and consistent with Takotsubo cardiomyopathy.

Recently, an association between significant MR and mitral valve tethering has been demonstrated in a subset of Takotsubo cardiomyopathy patients. In Takotsubo cardiomyopathy patients, SAM can also cause significant MR.

Reference

Izumo M, Nalawadi S, Shiota M, et al. Mechanisms of acute mitral regurgitation in patients with Takotsubo cardiomyopathy: an echocardiographic study. *Circ Cardiovasc Imaging.* 2011;4(4):392–398.

CASE 74

Respiratory Failure and Tachy-brady Syndrome

A 76-year-old woman had repeated hospital admissions for volume overload, respiratory failure, prolonged intubations, atrial fibrillation, and tachy-brady syndrome.

On repeated transthoracic echocardiograms (TTE), she has a normal to hyperdynamic left ventricular (LV) systolic function and variably moderate or severe pulmonary hypertension. She has difficult transthoracic images (Figs. 74-1 to 74-4 and Videos 74-1 and 74-2).

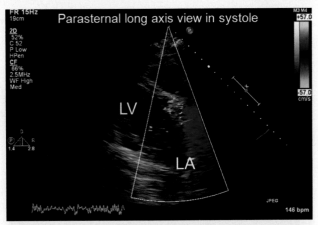

Figure 74-1.

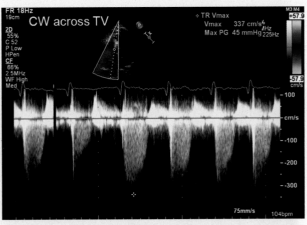

Figure 74-3.

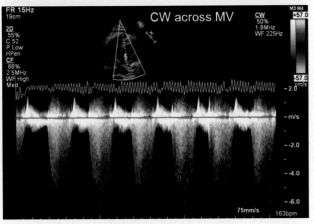

Figure 74-2.

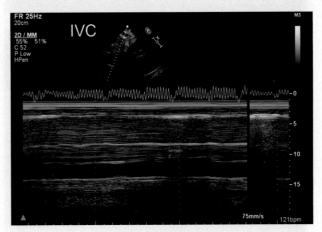

Figure 74-4.

QUESTION 1. Based on the findings, which test should be performed next?

- A. 12-lead electrocardiogram
- B. TTE with saline contrast
- C. Transesophageal echocardiogram (TEE)
- D. Cardiac catheterization

Answers

ANSWER 1: C. The transthoracic images are technically difficult. However, the 2D images (on video) demonstrate adequately hyperdynamic LV and right ventricular systolic function with a good tricuspid regurgitation signal and nice visualization of the inferior vena cava. Therefore, there would be no indication for either saline or LV contrast. However, although the color flow fails to demonstrate mitral regurgitation (MR), the continuous wave across the mitral valve clearly identifies MR, and the mitral E-inflow velocity is almost 1.5 m per second.

In a patient with poor image quality, normal LV ejection fraction, pulmonary hypertension, and repeated admissions for shortness of breath, significant MR needs to be considered, and a TEE would be indicated to better visualize the mitral valve (Fig. 74-5 and Videos 74-3 to 74-6).

The patient was indeed found to have severe MR by TEE, and she underwent successful percutaneous mitral valve repair.

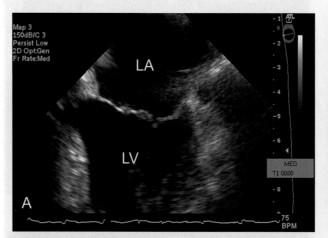

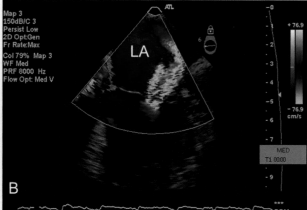

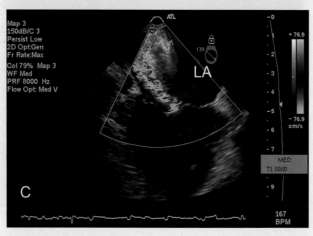

Figure 74-5. TEE four-chamber views (**A,B**); TEE two-chamber view (**C**).

Suggested Reading

Whitlow PL, Feldman T, Pedersen WR. Acute and 12-month results with catheter-based mitral valve leaflet repair: the EVEREST II (Endovascular Valve Edge-to-Edge Repair) High Risk Study. *J Am Coll Cardiol.* 2012;59:130–139.

CASE 75

Lung Cancer with Shortness of Breath

*T*his patient is an 83-year-old man with active lung cancer, and he was on chemotherapy. He had never had surgery and had never received radiation therapy.

He was referred to the emergency room for evaluation of shortness of breath. A transthoracic echocardiogram showed a possible vegetation of the aortic valve. A transesophageal echocardiogram (TEE) was performed to further evaluate the aortic valve.

See Figures 75-1 to 75-4 and Videos 75-1 to 75-4.

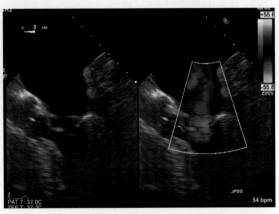

Figure 75-1.

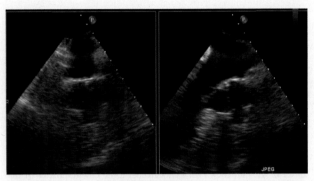

Figure 75-3.

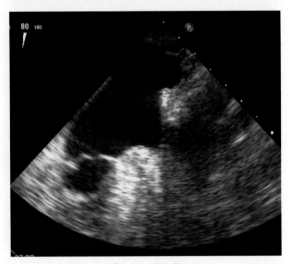

Figure 75-2.

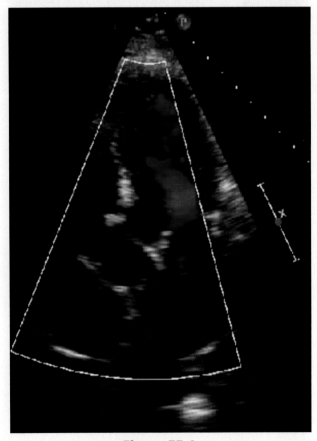

Figure 75-4.

QUESTION 1. Image quality of the TEE was not optimal. The reason for the low image quality TEE appeared to be a mass behind the left atrium. What is the next step to evaluate this mass?

A. Computed tomography (CT)/magnetic resonance imaging

B. Catheterization

C. Chest x-ray

D. Electrocardiogram

Answers

ANSWER 1: A. This patient has a history of lung cancer, and the mass appeared to be an extracardiac structure. A large hiatal hernia was detected by the CT scan (Fig. 75-5). The hiatal hernia was likely responsible for the poor image quality of the TEE.

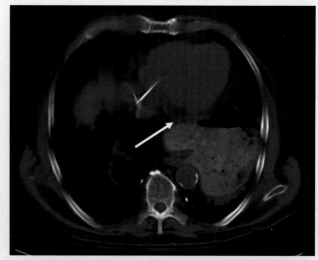

Figure 75-5.

Suggested Readings

D'Cruz IA, Hancock HL. Echocardiographic characteristics of dia-phragmatic hiatus hernia. *Am J Cardiol.* 1995;75:308–310.

Koskinas KC, Oikonomou K, Karapatsoudi E, et al. Echocardiographic manifestation of hiatus hernia simulating a left atrial mass: case report. *Cardiovasc Ultrasound.* 2008;6:46.

Clinical Findings and Echocardiographic Correlations

ECHO IMAGES

[Figs. A-J]

Echo A

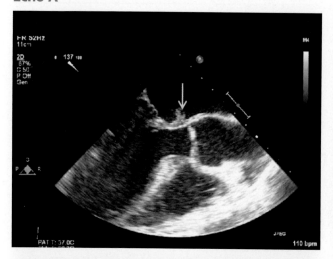

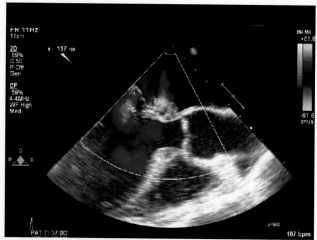

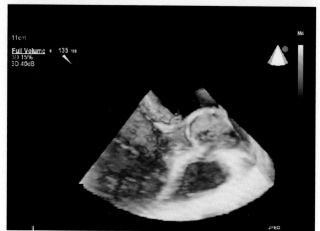

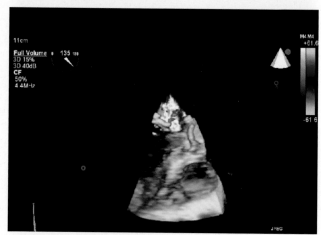

Echo B

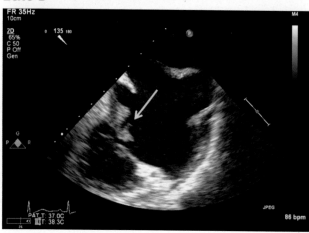

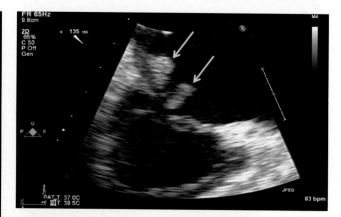

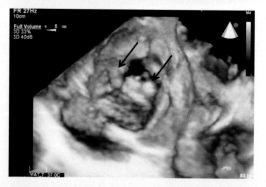

Case 5

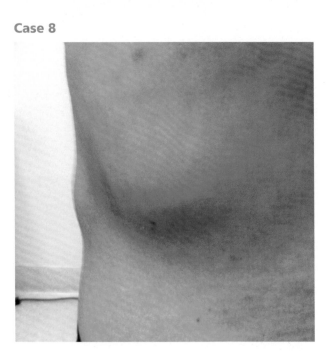

Case 6

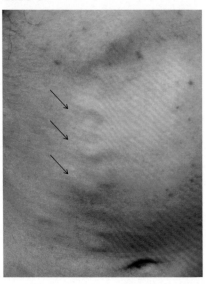

Case 7

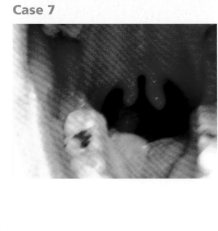

Case 8

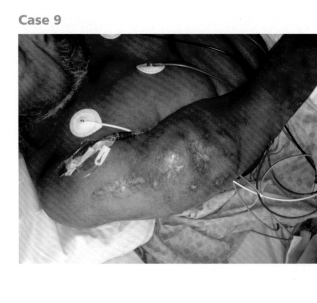

Case 9

Case 10

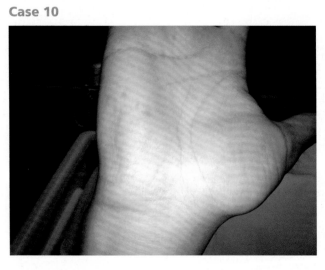

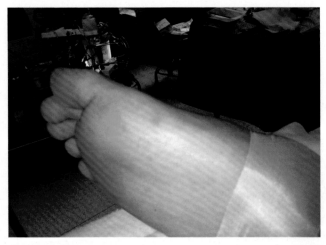

Match the physical finding images (Figs. 1-10) with the appropriate echo images (Figs. A-J).

PHYSICAL FINDINGS
[Figs. 1-10]

Case 1

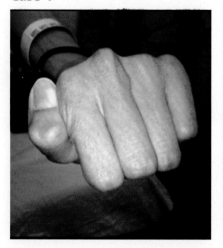
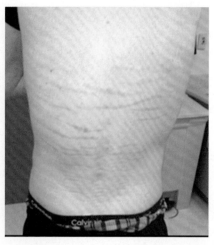
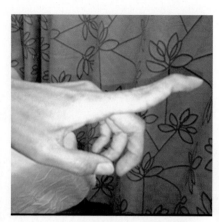

Case 2

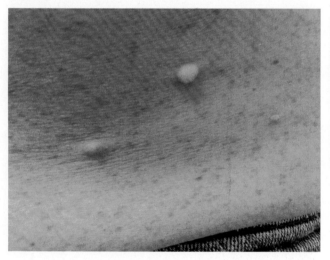
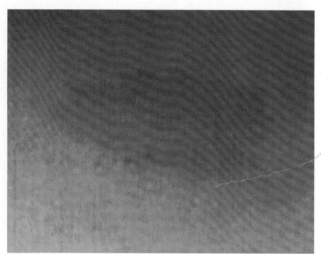

Case 3

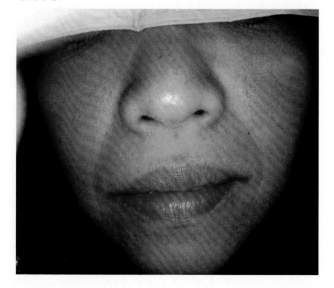

Case 4

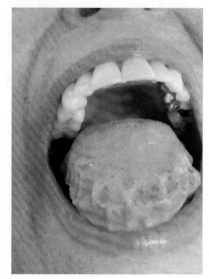

CASE 1

ANSWER 1: ECHO C. Clinical finding: Marfan syndrome. Picture shows arachnodactyly and skin striae that are typical musculoskeletal findings seen in Marfan syndrome. Marfan syndrome is an autosomal dominant condition (25% de novo) associated with mutations involving the Fibrillin 1 gene in most of the cases. (*Left panel*) Echocardiogram shows aortic root aneurysm with markedly dilated sinuses of Valsalva (*see arrows*), which are present in 60% to 80% of the patients and represents the main cause of morbidity and mortality among them (Hirata et al. *JACC* 1991). (*Right panel*) Image taken after aortic valve and root replacement with Bentall graft (Bentall et al. *Thorax* 1968).

CASE 2

ANSWER 2: ECHO E. Clinical finding: Neurofibromatosis (von Recklinghausen's disease). Picture shows classical cutaneous neurofibromas (*left*), freckles and café-au-lait spots (*right*) that are seen in neurofibromatosis (von Recklinghausen disease). The transthoracic echo shows findings consistent with hypertrophic cardiomyopathy, which has been associated to neurofibromatosis (Elliot et al. *Am Heart Jour.* 1976) possibly through a role of neurofibromin as a critical modulator or Ras protein activity in the cardiomyocytes (Xu et al. *Circ Res.* 2009).

CASE 3

ANSWER 3: ECHO D. Clinical finding. Rheumatic mitral stenosis. Mitral facies. Picture shows pinkish-purple malar flush, which can occur with rheumatic mitral stenosis. In many of these cases there is reduction in the cardiac output and severe pulmonary hypertension. Chronic hypoxemia produces vasoconstriction and livedo reticularis in the malar area (Blase et al. *Circulation* 2005). Echo shows rheumatic mitral stenosis (MS) (*arrow*) in 2D (*above*) or 3D echo (*below*). The main cause of MS, thought to be related to common M protein antigen between the heart and group A hemolytic *Streptococcus* resulting in an autoimmune attack after streptococcal infection. LA, left atrium; Ao, aorta; LV, left ventricle.

CASE 4

ANSWER 4: ECHO F. Clinical finding: Amyloidosis. Macroglossia (see teeth marks in the sides of tongue due to tongue enlargement causing the teeth to indent the lingual mucosa). A transthoracic echo shows findings consistent with amyloid. Namely, there is thickening of the left ventricular (LV) and right ventricular (RV) walls, and the myocardium appears bright. The deceleration time is short in the setting of thick LV walls, there is an "L" wave (*arrow*) indicating increased filling pressures as does the deceleration time and the ratio of E wave LV filling to the myocardial E' wave in diastole (E/E'). The small "s" wave (*asterisk*) on the tissue Doppler imaging is also indicative of poor contractile function. In amyloid there is replacement of normal myocardial contractile elements by infiltration of interstitial deposits of amyloid, leading to a firm, rubbery noncompliant (stiff) myocardium, most commonly caused by light-chain amyloidosis (Kushwaha et al. *NEJM* 1997). As a consequence of infiltration there is typically low voltage on the electrocardiogram (ECG). This then results in "voltage/mass discordance" with low-voltage on the ECG and poor R wave progression.

CASE 5

ANSWER 5: ECHO J. Clinical finding: Atheroemboli. Bluish discoloration of the fingers after cardiac catheterization. This phenomenon is known as blue-toe syndrome, as it occurs more frequently in the lower extremities. Echo shows aortic arch atherosclerotic plaque. Cholesterol crystal microemboli from the atherosclerotic plaque in a proximal large-caliber artery shower into the circulation occluding small arterioles, producing mechanical plugging and inflammation usually with an asymmetrical pattern (Falanga et al. *Arch Dermatol.* 1986). This usually coexists with livedo reticularis. Pulses usually remain palpable as lesions are in small arterioles.

CASE 6

ANSWER 6: ECHO G. Clinical finding: Caput medusa (*arrows*). Echo shows a large obstructive mass in the right atrium leading to markedly elevated central venous pressures. When portal hypertension occurs the umbilical vein, normally obliterated in early life, may re-open. This allows blood to be shunted through the periumbilical veins to the umbilical vein. In this case the lymphoma infiltrating the right atrium produces right-sided increased pressures leading to portal hypertension and portocaval shunt development.

CASE 7

ANSWER 7: ECHO H. Clinical finding: Loeys-Dietz syndrome. Picture shows a bifid uvula. Echo shows complex ascending aorta dissection (*yellow arrow*). Computed tomography shows cork screwing of the carotid arteries (*white arrows*). Loeys-Dietz syndrome is an autosomal dominant disorder caused by mutations in the genes encoding transforming growth factor beta receptor 1 and 2 (TGFBR1 or TGFBR2). De novo mutations represent 75% of cases and is typically characterized by the triad hypertelorism, cleft palate/bifid uvula, and/or arterial tortuosity. Early mortality is mainly due to aortic root dilatation leading to aortic dissection and rupture. It is recommended for these patients to have prophylactic aortic root replacement when the aortic root is 40 to 42 mm, earlier than Marfan patients' when prophylactic replacement is generally done at 50 mm. In addition, in Loeys-Dietz patients, vessels need to be screened from head to pelvis upon diagnosis (Van Hemelrijk et al. *Curr Opin Cardiol.* 2010).

CASE 8

ANSWER 8: ECHO I. Clinical finding: Metastatic liposarcomas in a patient. Picture shows that the patient has a subcutaneous mass in the back (liposarcoma). The echo shows a liposarcoma compressing the right ventricle. Liposarcoma is one of the most common soft-tissue malignant tumors. Myxoid variety represents 40% to 50% with primary location usually in the lower extremities. It can present as a primary heart lesion or as metastasis from a distal tumor. 2D echo is usually sufficient for diagnosis of cardiac involvement but magnetic resonance imaging may be considered for more comprehensive assessment of the tumor size, location, and tissue infiltration (Fairman et al. *Int Jour Cardiovasc Imag.* 2005).

CASE 9

ANSWER 9: ECHO B. Clinical finding: Right-sided infective endocarditis. Evidence of active and healing skin infections on the right arm due to intravenous drug abuse (IVDA) and skin injections. Echo shows multiple tricuspid valve vegetations (*marked with arrows*) in the 2D transthoracic echocardiogram (TTE) and 3D transesophageal echocardiogram (TEE). Infective endocarditis due to IVDA tends to be right-sided and more commonly associated with *Staphylococcus aureus*; though Streptococci, Enterococci and other organisms like fungi or gram-negative rods are also common. Usually it occurs in younger patients as compared to non-IVDA and produces more pulmonary emboli (Matthew et al. *Arch Intern Med.* 1995).

CASE 10

ANSWER 10: ECHO A. Clinical finding: Left-sided infective endocarditis. Picture shows multiple embolic lesions which are red and tender in the hands and feet of a patient with infective endocarditis. Echo shows vegetations, as well as perforation in the anterior mitral valve leaflet in 2D (*arrow*) and 3D TEE. We have found that 3D TEE is helpful in the diagnosis of valve perforations (Thompson et al. *Am J Cardiol.* 2010).

CASE 1

ANSWER 1. ECHO N. **Primum atrial septum defect/atrioventricular (AV) canal defect.** The electrocardiogram (ECG) shows first degree AV block and left-axis deviation (incomplete right bundle branch block [RBBB] and left anterior fascicular block). P-wave morphology suggests biatrial enlargement. The reasons for characteristic left-axis deviation in primum atrial septum defect (ASD) are not well understood but thought to be due to posterior AV node and bundle of His displacement due to an anterior unwedged aorta in respect to the mitral and tricuspid valve. The 2-dimensional echocardiogram (2D-echo) shows an atrioventricular canal defect with significant shunting and enlarged right and left atria (*a to c*). This condition is associated with Down syndrome patients (Web et al. *Circulation* 2006).

CASE 2

ANSWER 2. ECHO C. **Secundum atrial septum defect.** The ECG shows right-axis deviation and an incomplete RBBB. Right-axis deviation is due to right ventricular hypertrophy and strain due to pulmonary hypertension. The 2D echo shows an enlarged and hypertrophied right ventricle (RV) with marked right atrial (RA) enlargement. The echo lucency in the central portion of interatrial septum (IAS) suggests an atrial septum defect (ASD, *a*). An ASD with left to right shunting is confirmed by color Doppler in the 4-chamber (*b*) and subcostal views (*c*) and pulsed wave Doppler (*d*). Secundum ASD is more frequently found in females (Web et al. *Circulation* 2006).

CASE 3

ANSWER 3. ECHO D. **Stress-induced (Takotsubo) cardiomyopathy.** The initial ECG shows sinus tachycardia and is suspicious for acute myocardial ischemia/infarction (anterolateral leads). The 2D echo shows prominent left ventricular (LV) apical ballooning with preserved basal contractility (*a and b*). The changes on the follow-up ECG of T wave inversion in the precordial leads along with the echo findings support the diagnosis of stress induced (Takotsubo) cardiomyopathy. LV dysfunction is usually reversible, with low mortality, and good prognosis. This condition is more common in females and is often preceded by emotional or physical stress (Gianni et al. *Eur Heart J.* 2006).

CASE 4

ANSWER 4. ECHO G. **Ebstein's anomaly.** The ECG shows sinus tachycardia and a short PR interval on ECG. Close review of the QRS complex reveals delta waves. This type of pre-excitation pattern can be seen in up to 25% of patients with Ebstein's anomaly (mostly right posterior and right lateral accessory pathways). The 2D echo shows that the septal tricuspid leaflet insertion is displaced into the right ventricle (*a*, IAS: interatrial septum). Tricuspid valve coaptation is shifted apically and the right atrium ventricularized (*b*). Reduced RV volume and compliance and impaired tricuspid coaptation lead to severe TR and elevated right sided filling pressures. Consequently interatrial right to left shunting due to an ASD or a stretched persistent foramen ovale can occur frequently (Smith et al. *Am J Cardiol.* 1982; Sommer et al. *Circulation* 2008).

CASE 5

ANSWER 5. ECHO A. **Acute pulmonary embolism.** The ECG shows sinus tachycardia, RV strain and S1Q3T3 pattern (prominent S wave in lead I, a Q and inverted T wave in lead III). The 2D echo shows a dilated right ventricle (RV) with direct evidence for thrombus in transit in the RV (*a*) and right atrium (*b to c*) and the commonly observed pattern of mid-RV free wall hypokinesis, but preserved RV apical contractility (*c diastole versus d systole*). Termed McConnell's sign, this wall motion pattern has a low sensitivity but relatively high specificity in acute pulmonary embolism (Goldhaber. *The Lancet* 2004; McConnell et al. *Am J Cardiol.* 1996).

CASE 6

ANSWER 6. ECHO I. **Right ventricular hypertrophy.** The ECG shows complete heart block with occasional fusion beats, biatrial enlargement and a RBBB. Of significance are ECG signs for right axis deviation and right ventricular (RV) enlargement. The 2D echo shows a dilated RV (*a*) and significantly hypertrophied RV free wall of ~1 cm (*b*). In addition the right atrium is enlarged and the interatrial septum is bowing towards the left atrium suggesting elevated right-sided pressure compatible with significant underlying pulmonary hypertension (*b*) (Haddad et al. *Circulation* 2008).

QUIZ 2 ANSWERS

CASE 7

ANSWER 7. ECHO B. **Pericardial effusion.** The ECG is suspicious for low voltage. No alternating QRS axis can be observed but the magnitude of the ECG voltage varies from beat to beat. The additional ECG shows more exaggerated pattern of electrical alternans (courtesy of Dr. PK Shah). The 2D Echo shows a significant circumferential pericardial effusion (*a-c*) (Wann et al. *J Am Soc Echocardiography.* 2008).

CASE 8

ANSWER 8. ECHO F. **Aortic root abscess.** ECG recordings show interval development of complete AV block along with a right bundle branch block. The transesophageal echo reveals a thickened aortic root with varying ultrasound density (*a and b*). While such aortic root changes can be seen in the immediate postoperative AVR setting, they raise the suspicion of an aortic root abscess, which was confirmed at surgery in this patient (Brecker et al. *Heart.* 1999).

CASE 9

ANSWER 9. ECHO H. **Hypertrophic cardiomyopathy.** The ECG shows marked left ventricular (LV) hypertrophy and LV strain pattern. The sharply inverted T-waves in the precordial leads are typical for hypertrophic cardiomyopathy (HCM). The 2D echo shows marked symmetric LV wall hypertrophy. The combined ECG and echo findings in the absence of chronically elevated afterload (e.g. aortic stenosis, hypertension) and infiltrative cardiomyopathies make the diagnosis of HCM very likely (Wigle. *Heart.* 2001; Ho. *Circulation.* 2012).

CASE 10

ANSWER 10. ECHO M. **Amyloid heart disease.** The ECG shows limb lead low voltage and the 2D echo markedly increased left ventricular wall thickness (*a and b*). The combination of these findings suggests the diagnosis of amyloid heart disease. This echo further typically shows a thickened interatrial septum and small pericardial effusion (*a and b*). Diastolic filling shows a restricted pattern by mitral inflow Doppler (*c, lower panel*), an L-wave (*arrow*) indicative of elevated LV filling pressures and low myocardial velocities by tissue Doppler (*c, upper panel*). Commonly the myocardium looks characteristically sparkling and granular, but this appearance is not specific and exaggerated by today's harmonic imaging ultrasound technique (Dubrey et al. *Br J Cardiol.* 2009).

CASE 11

ANSWER 11. ECHO J. **Cardiac sarcoidosis.** The ECG shows sinus tachycardia with complete heart block and a junctional escape rhythm with repolarization abnormalities. Sarcoid granulomas in the myocardium can result in complete heart block (*as seen here*) as well has ventricular arrhythmias and mitral regurgitation when the granulomas involve the papillary muscles. The 2D echo shows a thinned interventricular basal septum (*arrow*), which was likely the site of a granuloma as the patient had angiographically normal coronary arteries. The echo also suggests left ventricular aneurysm formation (*a to c*). Nevertheless the echo has a low sensitivity and specificity to detect early cardiac sarcoidosis (Doughan et al. *Heart.* 2006).

CASE 12

ANSWER 12. ECHO K. **Apical hypertrophic cardiomyopathy: Yamaguchi syndrome.** The ECG shows marked left ventricular (LV) hypertrophy and deeply inverted T-waves in most of the limb and precordial leads. The 2D echo reveals predominantly apical left ventricular hypertrophy with a spade-like LV cavity (*a*). This was confirmed with ultrasound contrast opacifying the LV cavity in diastole (*b*) and systole (*c*). Yamaguchi Syndrome is a common, nonobstructive form of HCM in Japan, but much less commonly diagnosed in non-Asians (Yamaguchi et al. *Am J Cardiol.* 1979; Maron BJ. *JAMA* 2002).

CASE 13

ANSWER 13. ECHO E. **Chagas heart disease.** The ECG shows a right bundle branch and left anterior fascicular block, typical for the chronic Chagas disease stage. The 2D echo shows a LV apical aneurysm, which is often found in chronic Chagas-related heart disease. (*a and b*). Chagas disease is usually acquired in childhood and manifests in the acute phase as a febrile illness with rare cardiac involvement. Similar to this patient, patients present decades later in the chronic myocarditis Chagas disease stage and have ECG and echo findings as above (Acquatella. *Circulation* 2007).

CASE 14

ANSWER 14. ECHO L. **Ventricular fibrillation.** The ECG shows ventricular fibrillation. Echo M-mode shows no meaningful LV contraction and movement (*a*). The aortic valve does not open during systole (*b*). The 2D echo reveals an apical left ventricular assist device (LVAD) cannula with inflow into the LVAD confirmed by color Doppler (*c and d*) (Ammar et al. *Eur Heart J Cardiovasc Imaging.* 2012).

QUIZ 3 ANSWERS

CASE 1

ANSWER 1: B. For Case 1, the M-mode shows the classic flat E-F slope of the anterior mitral valve leaflet, lack of a-wave on the mitral leaflet, and the posterior leaflet moves in the same direction of the anterior leaflet, all of which are indicative of mitral stenosis. Figure B demonstrates an increased transmittal gradient (mean = 28 mm) and a flat deceleration time that are consistent with severe mitral stenosis.

CASE 2

ANSWER 2: A. For Case 2a, the M-mode shows random motion of the anterior leaflet in diastole as well as thickening of the posterior leaflet, which are suggestive of a flail mitral valve leaflet and possible vegetation. For Case 2b, the color M-mode corroborates significant mitral regurgitation seen as a blue signal in the left atrium throughout systole (during the entire time that the aortic valve is also noted to be open on the M-mode echo). The color Doppler also demonstrates some aortic regurgitation. Figure A1, the 2-D echo (four chamber view) shows a thickened mitral valve consistent with a vegetation as well as possible flail of the mitral leaflet. Figure A2, the same view with color Doppler, shows severe mitral regurgitation.

CASE 3

ANSWER 3: D. For Case 3, the M-mode echo shows systolic anterior motion (SAM) of the mitral valve with prolonged SAM–septal contact (consistent with a high left ventricular outflow tract [LVOT] gradient), and asymmetric septal hypertrophy and a small left ventricular cavity. These findings are typical of hypertrophic cardiomyopathy (HCM). Figure D shows an increased left ventricular outflow track gradient (92 mm Hg) which is late peaking (dagger shaped) and typical for HCM.

CASE 4

ANSWER 4: C. For Case 4, the M-mode through the anterior mitral leaflet demonstrates diastolic fluttering consistent with aortic regurgitation. Figure C demonstrates a continuous wave (CW) Doppler signal that is holodiastolic with a flat slope consistent with aortic regurgitation.

CASE 5

ANSWER 5: F. For Case 5, this M-mode is through the pulmonic valve and it demonstrates a loss of a-wave as well as a W-pattern which is indicative of severe pulmonary hypertension. Figure F shows the right ventricular outflow tract systolic flow signal. The time from onset to peak, known as the pulmonary acceleration time, is very short: 53 milliseconds. This is also consistent with severe pulmonary hypertension.

CASE 6

ANSWER 6: E. For Case 6, the M-mode echo through the mitral valve demonstrates late systolic mitral valve prolapse. The Doppler in E demonstrates late systolic mitral regurgitation.

CASE 7

ANSWER 7: H. For Case 7, the M-mode shows a very dilated right ventricle with paradoxical septal motion as timed on the electrocardiogram. These findings are consistent with right ventricular (RV) pressure and volume overload. Figure H1 shows severe tricuspid regurgitation (RV volume overload) and Figure H2 shows a CW Doppler signal with a RV to right atrial pressure gradient of 87 mm Hg indicative of RV pressure overload.

CASE 8

ANSWER 8: G. For Case 8, the M-Mode echo through the aortic valve shows aortic valve preclosure, which is a typical finding for discrete membranous subaortic stenosis (DSAS). Figure G shows an increase in LVOT gradient on CW Doppler with a morphology that is consistent with a fixed stenosis and in diastole there is evidence of aortic regurgitation. These findings are characteristic of DSAS in that the M-mode shows normal initial aortic cusp excursion before preclosure and the Doppler shows a high LVOT gradient associated with aortic regurgitation (common in DSAS).

CASE 9

ANSWER 9: J. For Case 9, the M-mode shows a small left and right ventricle, and there is only a trivial pericardial effusion anterior to the right ventricle. Clinically tamponade was suspected due to high central venous pressure and paradoxical pulse. Figure J1 shows Doppler mitral inflow variation consistent with tamponade. Figure J2 shows no significant pericardial effusion but very large and bilateral pleural effusions which in this case are the cause of clinical, hemodynamic, and Doppler findings of tamponade.

CASE 10

ANSWER 10: I. For Case 10, the color M-mode shows findings indicative of both significant aortic and mitral regurgitation. The 2D echo image in Figure I1 shows a flail and perforated anterior mitral leaflet as well as aortic valve vegetation. Figure I2 shows severe aortic regurgitation as well as diastolic mitral regurgitation.

INDEX